Your Looks

Younger & Better

Through Cosmetic Surgery

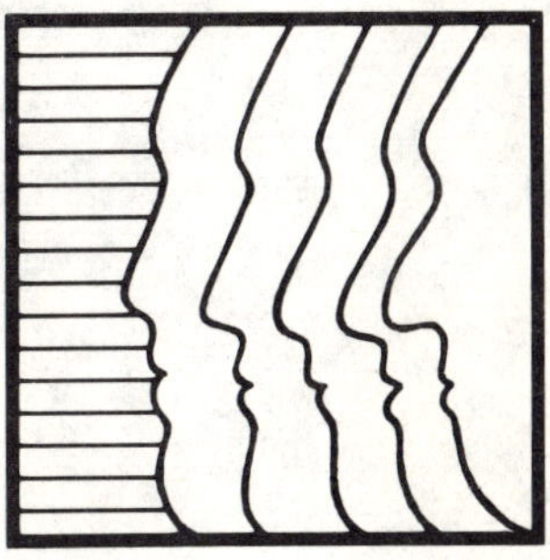

To Deborah
my best wishes —
R B Creasonwell
Sept '82

Your Looks

Younger & Better

Through Cosmetic Surgery

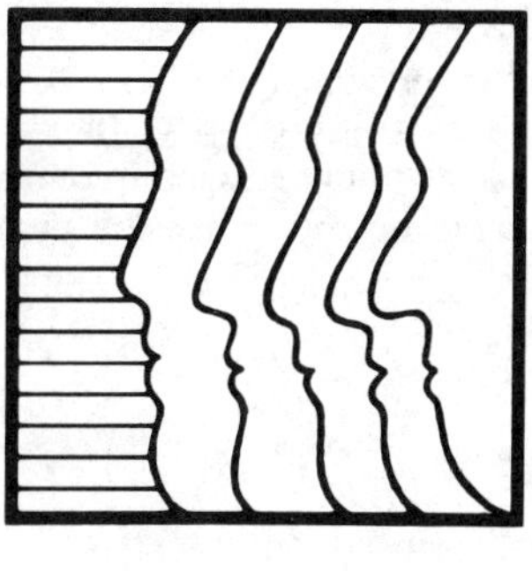

by

Richard B. Aronsohn, MD.

NURSECO, Inc.

Pacific Palisades, California

NURSECO, Inc.
PO Box 145
Pacific Palisades, CA. 90272

Library of Congress Cataloging in Publication Data

Aronsohn, Richard B. 1926-
Your looks.

Includes index.
1. Surgery, Plastic. I. Title.
RD119.A76 617'.95 80-28618
ISBN 0-935236-17-1

Printed in the United States of America

Designed by Robert Liljenwall

Contents

Preface: 1981

The appalling human devastation of World War I was the catalyst for the rapid advancement of plastic surgery, which had, up to that time, developed in a rather desultory fashion. The knowledge and possibilities opened up to army doctors trying to repair torn young bodies were brought into vivid practice in World War II. The amazing surgical achievements on victims of that second conflict served to advance aesthetic techniques and pave the way toward cosmetic surgery, which had hitherto been wrapped in a haze of romanticism, mysticism, and special interests. Until not too long ago "beauty surgery" remained cloaked in mystery, with both surgeons and their patients appearing as shadowy figures; it is only in the last decade that aesthetic surgery has become a fully recognized specialty in its own right.

Along the way, a gullible public has accumulated a wealth of erroneous conceptions and preconceptions about the potential powers of cosmetic surgery. Many actually believe in miracle transformations of appearance comparable to the amazing cures achieved by wonder drugs and touted by the broadcast and publishing media. There are some who believe that a feature can be altered with little effort and without a convalescent period—that cosmetic surgery somehow surpasses conventional surgery. I hope to dispel such naive notions. Yet, in a very real sense this surgery does go beyond more orthodox operations. It is more than the embellishment of the surface; it is a door opened onto the psyche. In the combined psychological and aesthetic sense, the change can be near-miraculous. If so, the miracle lies within the artistry and skill of the attending surgeon.

In a way of speaking, the cosmetic surgeon is both architect and artist, for he designs on living canvas and carves from human flesh. Such skills should be available to those who set a prize, if not a price, on their appearance.

What are the merits of cosmetic surgery, its limitations, and potential hazards? How much does it cost? Is hospitalization necessary and is there much discomfort? How do I find a competent cosmetic surgeon? These are some of the questions that people considering this kind of surgery ask. To my knowledge, this book answers virtually every relevant concern raised by the potential patient.

About 90 percent of all cosmetic surgery concerns the head and neck. About 90 percent of this book is addressed toward that area. Therefore the emphasis and sequence of cosmetic operations follow those encountered in the surgeon's practice. Many of the ideas expressed on such matters as surgical technique and postoperative care convey varying viewpoints. Surgery, like medicine, is an inexact art and operative techniques and patient care may vary among surgeons, depending upon their individual judgment, skill, and experience. Two physicians may be equally learned, equally skilled, equally competent, but there may still be a disparity in their methods of operation based on different approaches. However, the surgical result is really what matters and it is not important if different approaches lead to the same cosmetic end. Along with techniques, fees also vary among surgeons. For each procedure, I present a range of prevailing rates.

Throughout the book, the personal pronouns he and she, and their variations, are used and are, of course, interchangeable. However, the reader will readily observe that the feminine pronoun predominates when I refer to patients. Although vanity and the urge for self-preservation are not the exclusive domain of women, it is a documented and undisputed fact that cosmetic surgery serves more women than men. Conversely, although there are female cosmetic surgeons, most practitioners of this art are men.

What I have to say is an essence of views distilled out of twenty-two years' experience in cosmetic surgery. They are melded into this book into whose pages, therefore, a prodigious amount of information has been injected. The prospective patient has here a rich lode of cosmetic ore for I have mined and filtered material previously obtainable only in surgical journals. My goal has been to impart accurate knowledge with precise language. The reader, however, need swallow no indigestible chunks of anatomical detail for I have translated medical terminology into understandable, easy reading.

In the last analysis, it is the photographs that tell the tale. Without one word of text, the pictures throughout this book can illustrate the benefit of cosmetic surgery to all who are interested in retaining youth and achieving beauty.

There are many people who deserve mention for the emergence and publication of this book. I would like to thank my patients who donated the pre- and postoperative photos shown throughout the book. Their willingness to display their before and after pictures demonstrates the maturity that cosmetic surgery has attained in the psychology of self-improvement.

To my office staff, Cathy, Evelyn, and Grace, for their patience and help, particularly in obtaining consents, photographs, and identification of patients.

To my publishers at Nurseco, Margo Neal and Edward Provenzano, for their constructive ideas which helped make the book even more interesting and understandable.

And to my wife, Valerie, whose insistence that I write this book is the sole reason for its existence. Her emotional and literary assistance throughout the planning and writing of these pages were invaluable to me. This text is dedicated to her.

Richard B. Aronsohn, MD
Los Angeles, California
1981

Foreword

As a psychotherapist, I am continually in touch with the emotional problems of people and from my personal experience, I know that not all forms of neuroses result from basic personality disturbances. Many emotional problems are realistic responses to external situations and social pressures.

Consider how inadequate an aging adult is made to feel if he or she is not young looking, because in the crowded and fiercely competitive marketplace, being old and looking it can be a real impediment. Obsolescence comes early. A job lost today at 40 or 45 may be the last job.

Or consider how different and even ugly a child may feel when burdened with a large and unattractive nose. This could have a negative effect on that child's development and his ability to relate to his peers. These children grow up to be adults who are saddened by the characteristics in their appearance that they feel are aberrant, and carry on through life as depressed and unhappy individuals.

How unnecessary!

My work is helping people to feel good about themselves; to enhance their self-esteem and self-respect; to expand their social and work skills; and generally to develop their total personalities.

While my major thrust concerns intense concentration on working from the inside out, with each client I do even more. That is, I encourage them to work from the outside in. And this is where the artistic talent of the cosmetic surgeon can help enrich a personality.

Fortunately, in this era of technological advancements where man is miraculously conquering space, other technological advances in the field of cosmetic surgery seem equally miraculous. Part of my routine as a therapist is often to encourage clients to seek the aid and advice of a cosmetic surgeon. During a session, I frequently pick up the phone and call experts such as Dr. Richard Aronsohn to get information about some particular feature or physical defect that might be troubling my client.

Many of you do not have the advantage of being able to dial a friend and receive the details you'll need about a particular aesthetic problem. Happily, you now have the advantage of referring to this thorough book, which offers the kind of honest, reliable, and accurate information you will require to make those important decisions about your life.

Why not look and feel more beautiful? Why not look younger and feel wonderful? You deserve the best and I want you to have it. Read on and find out how cosmetic surgery can positively influence your life.

Dr. Irene Kassorla

Dr. Irene Kassorla is a psychotherapist and author of two best-selling books, "Putting It All Together" (Warner Books) and "Nice Girls Do" (Stratford Press).

1
Of Ugly Ducklings and Beautiful Swans

It may well be true that beauty is only skin deep, but no culture (at least not yet) has proposed the slogan "Ugliness is only skin deep." The aphorism suggests that either we rarely look beyond the skin or we debase the true value of beauty to rationalize the squalor beneath the surface of life. Beauty may indeed be only skin deep but, failing X-ray vision, what else can we see?

Although beauty has always been a marvelous asset and a delight to the eye, social scientists once led us to believe that it was a very superficial quality, one having little influence on most people's lives. Recent research, however, suggests that physical attractiveness carries greater impact than previously suggested, and its influence begins startlingly early.

Growing Up With Cinderella

So early, in fact, that by the time we are toddlers, aesthetic standards are ingrained within us. We learn to identify beauty with goodness and ugliness with evil. Many fairy tales are told of the princess beautiful beyond reality and of the ugly witch who mistreats her. The prince who rescues the dazzling maiden from the ugly old witch is always handsome beyond belief. Thus, beauty is woven into the fabric of childhood fantasy. For the youth who cannot cope with his appearance, the fable of the ugly duckling lends hope that redemption is possible through cosmetic surgery.

Dreams of beauty continue beyond childhood. We live in a society that reveres youth and physical attractiveness. For all our talk about inner values and character, we tend to assume the best about attractive people. We are truly a skin-deep society—what we see is what we believe. Beauty colors our thinking when we first meet people for we are wedded to our eyes when it comes to first impressions.* Physical attractiveness goes a long way and is a crucial standard in our initial judging of people. It lands us jobs, gets officials elected, and is probably the single most important criterion in determining one's popularity in the late teens and early twenties.

Beauty Is . . . Is . . . Is . . .

Attempts to define beauty are mostly philosophical exercises. Why a beautiful face is beautiful remains a veiled subject. Yet, if beauty cannot be skewered mathematically, uncomeliness is readily perceived. Whatever the definition, craving for beauty and adornment, and the response to them, are older than recorded history. Anthropologists suggest that the urge for beautifying ourselves emerged when the human animal evolved into a thinking being and first saw his face reflected from water.

Whatever stands as the epitome of beauty, the wish to be beautiful lies within us all. To paraphrase an old cliche, behind every unattractive woman lurks a beauty pleading to be let out. For a fortunate few, the plea is unneeded for the wish is granted at birth. For most of us, backbone serves better than wishbone; an illusion of comeliness is attainable through ingenuity, diligence, and artful cosmetics. Beauty requires time, discipline, and money. We must work at it, and even those gifted with it must toil to retain it. Beauty demands practical routines—time necessary to attain, maintain, and sustain an attractive appearance. Although homeliness can be forever, without painstaking effort, beauty soon fades.

Mirror, Mirror On the Wall

Appearance is especially important to women in a way that men do not experience. There are persistent and pervasive forms of employment discrimination in this country against the plain-looking woman. Men face no such prejudice, except possibly in the cinema and politics. What makes this discrimination so treacherous is that few will admit that it exists. What employer in his right mind will tell a woman that he cannot hire her because she is unattractive and what woman meeting such bias is likely to publicize it. Female applicants must be able, capable, young, and attractive. What many employers really want is a woman with

**Rarely does one get a second chance to make a good first impression.*

thirty years' experience who looks twenty-five.

More than a generation ago, many women shied away from using rouge, nail polish, and other cosmetics. Those who did not were generally marked as "fast." Today hardly any woman shuns makeup. Hairpieces, facials, massages, mud and mineral baths, hormone and rejuvenation creams, youth pills, and cosmetics (for both men and women) are being bought in staggering quantities. It all comprises an expensive and somehow frantic pursuit of youth and beauty. In the United States, cosmetics and other beautifiers constitute an annual multibillion dollar industry.

It is an industry that transcends economic swings, for beauty knows no recession. Women know that a beautiful face is a strong if silent recommendation. A pretty woman, much less a beautiful one, isn't apt to suffer or go hungry. Beauty is a commodity that throughout history has always been in demand; indeed, occasionally it has changed the course of history.

With persuasive advertisements and cunning repetition, both men and women are pressured to improve their appearance. The unrelenting message suggests that they have only to invest in a few strategic cosmetics to acquire the irresistible allure of a Tahitian princess, the glamor of a celebrated star. By using the products publicized, it is hinted, not only will a woman keep her spouse from straying, but likely she will also require armed guards to ward off impassioned admirers, while a man will have his pick of ardent women. However, reality ultimately intrudes, if not to the eyes of the consumers, then to those who observe them.

The quest for beauty has always been restricted by the availability of medical and cosmetic aids. We can imagine the Queen of Sheba primping with scents, pigments, and oils, but never dreaming of a rhinoplasty. Salome could order cosmetics, adornments, even a severed head, but she could not command a face-lift. Millions of women, from the biblical era to the twentieth century, have yearned for a beauty potion. Only in the last three decades has cosmetic plastic surgery matured—to where it offers queen and average woman alike a tonic, if not an elixir. To succeed in the quest for youth and beauty, more and more men and women are turning to the cosmetic surgeon.

Beauty Surgery . . . It's Just a Cut Above

Two well-defined branches of corrective surgery have evolved which, although separated by title, often occupy the same shelf. General plastic surgery is a specialized branch of reparative surgery that embodies certain artistic principles in an effort to improve or restore the function, physiology, or appearance of an organ. This field has spawned a new breed of specialists who devote their entire practice to procedures with an aesthetic goal. They are called cosmetic surgeons. Plastic surgery concerns itself with the restoration of an organ and the possible improvement of appearance. Cosmetic surgery endeavors to improve appearance without interfering with function. Although there is a cosmetic component in plastic surgery and a reconstructive component in cosmetic surgery, they differ slightly in that one strives for normalcy, the other for beauty.

It takes talent and ingenuity to renovate an old face, so the practitioner of this new specialty must possess a unique combination of skill and artistry. He must pay attention and give time and effort to the smallest of details in surgery. This extra care quite often separates a good result from a poor one. He must also have profound emotional insight, for his incisions may be more than skin-deep—they can slice deep into the psyche as well. For each ripple of change upon the surface, there may be a torrential backlash on the patient's psychological makeup and emotional behavior. Unlike other surgeries, the cosmetic surgeon's handiwork, good or bad, is always on display.

A psychological filter ought to be built into a cosmetic surgeon's brain, for in essence he must be a surgical psychiatrist; indeed, he is unique in his ability to achieve psychotherapy through a scalpel. Aesthetic surgery, although often physiologically unnecessary, at times can be psychologically essential.

Cosmetic Surgery in the Eighties

Although cosmetic surgery is not a new art, it has only recently approached a high level of competence and recognition. Just as in the past the average person's aversion toward mental illness hampered psychiatry for many years, a peculiar attitude toward people who desired aesthetic surgery, and to the physicians who performed it, hindered the emergence of this specialty from medicine's shadow world. It was acceptable to have hair styled any which way or colored any hue; cosmetics elicited even less gossip and who was ever criticized for joining a gym in an effort to improve a bulging figure; but commit yourself to surgery in order to correct a defect that no cosmetic could hide, and you were suddenly denounced for "tampering with God's handiwork" or labeled as vain or narcissistic. Even physicians did not escape the prejudice. Saving lives, alleviating pain, and preventing and curing diseases have always been seen as the mission of the physician. The concept of surgery for the improvement of facial appearance was more difficult to accept. It simply was not respectable and was held in low esteem by the renowned surgeons of the day.*

Attitudes, however, change. What was once considered a hush-hush matter, beyond the pale of ethical surgery, has now gained widespread acceptance and even status. No one need apologize, feel vain, selfish, or stigmatized for wanting to improve his appearance or self-esteem. Many patients feel guilty and embarrassed about their apparent narcissism and need to be reassured that the desire for physical attractiveness is rational and normal. It is not vanity to correct a flaw; it is negligence not to.

No One's Perfect

As an artisan, nature is not always flawless. A pretty or handsome face often hovers in the shadow of a single ugly feature that asserts its domination. Large, limpid eyes are easily obscured by a twisted nose. A neat and shapely head can be marred by oversized, protruding ears. In life's game of chance, luck is often lost in the genes. But the roll of the dice need not be irrevocable. Cosmetic plastic surgery can correct the erratic growth of bone and cartilage; often it can accomplish much more.

Facial deformities, in particular, are the most difficult to bear. Psychologically the face is preeminent among the body parts, for it is the most visible and expressive in relation to the others and it is continually exposed to the ruthless scrutiny of our fellow beings. A disfigurement need not be glaring, just large enough to draw attention and comment. Thus, facial asymmetries and deformities constitute over 90 percent of all cosmetic surgery. As we cover less and visualize more, the rest of the body is also becoming a candidate for remodeling.

You learn rather quickly, if you are the surgeon, that the size of the deformity bears little relationship to the anxiety it produces. The ratio of "degree of deformity to intensity of

**Cosmetic surgeons were at first relegated to social infamy; only a few brave, well-trained doctors ventured into this specialty. This allowed many unqualified "practitioners" to exploit those who sought help for their deformities.*

feeling" is a very critical one. What may be trivial to one individual can be of tremendous significance to someone else. Even if relatively minor, a person's sense of deformity can be overwhelming to himself if not to others.

The Psychological Factor

Many young persons are convinced that they are unattractive because their features do not measure up to those of the currently reigning actor or actress or some other idol whom they worship. These fancied deformities can be just as debilitating as physical ones. Since the dividing line between a real disfigurement and an imaginary one is often blurred, the careful psychological evaluation and handling of a patient are more necessary in cosmetic surgery than in any other surgical specialty.

Those desiring cosmetic operations are often labelled as neurotic. Quite the contrary! Experience in dealing with thousands of such patients indicates that these individuals base their desire for an improved appearance on sound, tangible reasons. They may lack confidence because of self-consciousness due to an oversized nose, a receded chin, or some other physical abnormality; or feeling inwardly young, may want to project that vibrancy to others. They may fear that they cannot inspire love or recognition because of their looks and frequently are unable to give of themselves because the feeling of not having a chance blocks their capacity for trying. They may dream of beauty, but their dreams are imprisoned in reality.

Therapists have discovered that appearance outside the accepted norm can draw as much criticism from the community as deviant behavior does. The individual with a physically crippling disability or illness such as heart disease, paralysis, a missing limb, or blindness often cannot conform, but he is usually accorded attendant sympathy and extra consideration. People may even be impressed by how well such a person manages. He is more apt to accept his handicap than someone with a disfigurement because it is the disability, not society, that limits his activity.

Those with aesthetic deformities, on the other hand, soon become aware of hostile social attitudes. Regarded and treated differently, they imagine they are different and may develop a negative self-image, thereby further isolating themselves from society. These individuals live under a blanket of grief, always comparing themselves unfavorably with others. Such preoccupation can become so firmly entrenched that it warps the person's emotional health and often leads to physical disorders. Though beauty may be skin deep, the sense of one's ugliness sinks deeper, destroying the spirit and stunting a person's emotional life as well as inducing physical illness. Without exaggeration, ugliness can be called a disease, causing torment of body and soul. It is natural and sensible to try to eradicate that disease with a cosmetic cure.

The Decision

The person who consults the cosmetic surgeon differs from the usual patient in that he seeks an operation, whereas the other confers reluctantly with a general surgeon, hoping that an operation is unnecessary. Unlike general surgery, the need for cosmetic surgery does not carry, by today's standards, the special status of being ill. Illness forces acceptance of both immediate risks of surgery and its subsequent complications. The philosophy of cosmetic surgery is quite different. The patient is either well or in a relatively good medical state, and he hopes to gain a maximum of improvement with a minimum of risk. The patient concerned about his appearance usually thinks of himself not as sick but as homely or "deformed", a state sometimes equated with being morally "bad" or incapable of inspiring love. Thus, the aesthetic surgeon takes a well person and makes him sick for a while in an effort to improve him. If the transformation does not live up to the patient's expectations, it can be shattering, with the possible mushrooming of a neurosis already lurking within the person's unhappiness with the misshapen feature. Both suicide attempts and assaults on the surgeon have been recorded.

The cosmetic surgeon therefore must never permit his point of view to be restricted to just the patient's defect. He must develop a broader perspective and remember that there is a sensitive person attached to that feature. It does not make any difference whether or not the surgeon believes that surgery is important as long as the patient believes that it is. Thus, the doctor must treat the patient and not merely the local disfigurement. The patient's mental state is of crucial import, for it is his emotional temper that permits him, in full knowledge of the discomfort and risks, to submit to an elective operation.

For the patient, a cosmetic operation may be a monumental experience. Although the technical aspects of a surgical procedure may be "old hat" in the surgeon's eyes, the operation is new to the patient. Psychologically, minor surgery is a major event. The conscientious surgeon will respect it as such.

Expectations Sometimes Get in the Way

Often the success of surgery depends upon the change that the patient envisioned beforehand. Surgical results which are perfect successes in some people's estimation may appear failures to others. In general, adolescents are likely to have good results because their self-identity is still formative and physical changes are accordingly easier to integrate into their own concept of their body type. Older individuals, on the other hand, are apt to have long-standing disfigurements that often have set up personality barriers, thus inhibiting the pleasure or even the acknowledgment of any aesthetic improvement.

Some who undergo cosmetic surgery hope for a restoration of their youth, the reconstruction of an inadequate personality, the salvation of a shaky marriage, the rekindling of a cooling love affair. What they fail to realize is that no amount of surgery can bring about a rebirth or change the way a husband or wife sees their spouse. In television and movies they watch the miraculous metamorphosis of a human scarecrow into a swanlike beauty. They are certain that such transformations are commonplace and are stunned when the effect of their surgery is not as dramatic. While remarkable alterations are possible, the degree of success achieved is, more often than not, dependent upon the original material that one was given to work with. Although the surgeon can be a seeming wizard with the scalpel, he is a physician, not a magician.

Improvement, not perfection, is the goal of cosmetic surgery. Few results are miraculous, some are spectacular, but the majority involve subtle improvements in appearance. An unqualified success cannot be expected from every operation. Any surgery entails the possibility of complications since there is an intrinsic risk of failure in all operations. Not only are we dealing with living tissue, but the capricious healing process of that tissue lends its own personal touch to surgery. Although one strives for perfection during surgery, to expect it in every case is unrealistic. The surgeon who rigidly demands nothing less can end up on the psychiatric couch.

Self-Image . . . It's Just Your Point of View

Not all unattractive people request cosmetic surgery. Some with marked disfigurements that could be readily improved suffer little or no mental distress. Others who have had their abnormalities corrected still cherish their neuroses over these features just as if they had never been altered. Why do individuals with normal, or at least acceptable, faces have psychological problems over their features and react as if they had an actual disfigurement? In the shifting sands of beauty, self-image and its attendant psychology is the cornerstone upon which the rock of cosmetic surgery is based.

We emerge from childhood with certain convictions about ourselves—convictions for the most part submerged in our unconsciousness. Whether or not we realize it, each of us is invested with a mental picture of ourselves. This self-image is our own conception of the sort of person we are and what we imagine we look like. It is the sum of our past experiences, successes, failures, our belief in ourselves, and the way people have reacted and continue to react to us. Self-image is the key to personality and behavior and is fundamental in our personal adjustment to the world we live in. Psychologists have shown that it's really not important what the other person thinks of you, or what he thinks you look like. What is important is what you think he thinks of you and what you think he thinks you look like. Status and appearance matter primarily to oneself.

To have peace of mind and to find life reasonably satisfying, each of us must have an adequate and realistic self-image that we can live with—a picture of self that is acceptable to us. Cosmetic surgery can expand a stunted self-image, for personality enrichment following successful surgery occurs much too frequently to be merely coincidental. Some individuals undergo effective surgery yet continue to wear the same old personality. In these cases, their image of themselves is so impoverished that only psychotherapy can help.

"Women are as old as they look; men are as old as they feel." Because our society measures the sexes in that way, a greater number of women undergo cosmetic corrections. However, this surgery now beckons alluringly to the male. This increased interest has been generated mainly by the female's acceptance of the surgery. Increasingly women are urging their husbands or boyfriends to enhance their looks. Interestingly enough, surgeons find that men can be as vain as women; they are only less vocal and honest about it. Most women admit that their image is less than ideal; most men do not. In addition, it is difficult for some men to undergo the cosmetic operation for acceptance may signify to them that they are effeminate.

The desire for cosmetic surgery can render an individual peculiarly vulnerable since those whose commercial interest exceeds their professional skill may prey upon her eagerness. Never leap into cosmetic surgery before looking into it thoroughly. Because of the mystical aura that still surrounds this field, many people have fallen into the hands of charlatans or technicians with little experience or training. When the surgeon is highly competent, his price may be high; however, surgery works best with the best doctor and cut-rate surgery is catastrophic at any price.

The Bottom-Line—Choosing the Surgeon

How do you find a competent surgeon? One way is referral by a friend or acquaintance who has undergone successful surgery. Another is to ask your personal physician. Or you can call the local county medical society. But it is a clerk employed by the society who answers the phone. He punches a computer containing a list of qualified surgeons who are registered and recommends several who are next up for referral; although they may be adequate, they may not be the most competent. To solve this dilemma, consult several of these surgeons. Inquire as to how many successful cases each has performed. This is important. Years of experience can be misleading. In practicing his craft, the artisan may have performed the surgery in question only once a year for twenty years—yet can boast of twenty years' experience. If necessary, ask the surgeon about his specialty training, and when in his office, look for specialty training degrees. These do not guarantee a successful operation nor a good result, but do demonstrate that he has had specific preparation in this field, a field where without artistry, skill, and rigorous training, he can be a menace in the operating theater.

The validation of any surgical procedure is the happiness and improved well-being derived from it. The increasing demand for aesthetic surgery is ample proof of its acceptance. Each year more than a million people undergo elective surgery to improve their appearance—and there is no end in sight. If it can be labeled a luxury, cosmetic surgery is the cheapest one today. The middle-aged woman who saves up to buy a $10,000 fur coat would probably be happier with a $3500 face-lift.

In the future, we may well view the correction of disfigurements by a cosmetic surgeon as casually as a visit to the hairdresser. However, basic aesthetic improvement will probably provide more substantial benefits than a new hairdo.

When asked her secret to beauty, a famous movie actress once replied, "I don't drink, I don't smoke, I don't stay up late, and—I've got a fabulous cosmetic surgeon!" Most likely these habits would not apply to all of us, but like our movie stars, we all would like to stay young and be beautiful. To fulfill that desire, the cosmetic surgeon comes closest, in reality, to a fairy godmother. He alone can change an ugly duckling into a beautiful swan.

Q&A

What are the background and training of a cosmetic surgeon? Do they include training in art and psychology?

At the present time, educational programs teach the techniques of plastic surgery; no residency (training) program in cosmetic surgery exists. The art of aesthetic surgery and its attendant psychology are acquired in one's practice. This is a valid reason for seeking an experienced surgeon to perform one's surgery.

Is cosmetic surgery available everywhere in the United States?

Although cosmetic surgery is performed throughout the United States, the highest incidence (and the predominance of specialists in the field) is centered in New York, Los Angeles, and Miami. Some patients believe that they must travel to Europe or South America for their operation. The fact is that the best cosmetic surgery in the world is performed in the United States.

Do other cultures practice what you would consider a form of cosmetic surgery?

Certain tribal Africans are recognized by their characteristic alterations of the human body. Without question, their scarification of the body, distortion of lips and ears, and thrusting of bones or ivory through the nostrils are a form of cosmetic surgery, bizarre as these may seem to us.

What is the best way to find the most capable cosmetic surgeon to correct a facial deformity that I have?

At present, there are several types of specialists who perform cosmetic surgery of the face and neck: dermatologists, ophthalmologists, general plastic surgeons, head and neck surgeons, and ear, nose, and throat specialists. No one of these specialists has a monopoly in the field no matter what you may have read. Among each group are those who are more gifted, talented, and artistic. These individuals will generate the best results in the greatest percentage of cases. It is to be hoped that you will be referred to one of these by another satisifed patient. As indicated earlier in the chapter, your private physician can also refer you to a capable surgeon. The knowledge of who is doing very good work gets around in medical circles. Aside from that, you can inquire of your local county medical society, which will recommend several surgeons. You must now make a decision after consulting with one or all of the physicians recommended. It can be difficult. Your "gut" feeling quite often makes the decision for you.

My friends think that I am vain and silly to have my nose corrected. Should I feel embarrassed about wanting to fix my nose?

Certainly not. To improve your self-esteem and quality of life is a very positive and rational move. It is far better to take constructive, bold action about a problem than to brood and worry about it while doing nothing. There is no harm in listening to what your friends have to say, but each of us must take charge of our own life and do what is best for us.

2
The Nose—Give It A Break

Some girls insist on fancy cars,
Like Cadillacs and sleek Jaguars;
Or they want men with Swiss chateaux.
All I want is a pretty nose.

REFRAIN:
  A pretty nose,
  A pretty nose—
  Not Tiffany jewels or Dior clothes
  Or crowns of gold or lace trousseaux
  Are nicer than a pretty nose.

Some ask for yachts and diamond rings
And ever more expensive things
To satisfy their quid-pro-quos.
But I'm all yours for a pretty nose.

An awful lot of gals want furs
And walk-in wardrobes all marked "hers."
For me no frills and furbelows—
Just serve me up a pretty nose.

Now that's not much to ask, I think.
It isn't gold; it isn't mink,
Or a thousand pair of nylon hose,
Or tickets to the Broadway shows,
Or French maids standing by in rows—
But just a nicer, neat and straighter
More attractive
Nose!

—R. B. Aronsohn, M.D.

The most common operation performed by the cosmetic surgeon is a rhinoplasty, or nose correction. Residing as it does in the center of the face in both the vertical and horizontal planes, the nose is the focal point of the face. Architecturally, more than any other feature, the nose unifies the face, and psychologically, our emotions quite often focus on it.

Functionally Speaking

Since breathing can be accomplished through the mouth and smelling has declined to merely a secondary role, the importance of the nose might be challenged. Yet it shows no inclination for following the little toe into extinction. From an evolutionary standpoint, the original function of the nose was primarily smelling—smelling for the detection of food and potential enemies. The respiratory process was added long after the origin of animal life. No longer do we depend upon smell rather than sight for recognition of the opposite sex (as do animals); we must now sniff to smell rather than breathe to smell. However, as the sense of smell has diminished with the passage of time, cultural pressures have forged another role for the nose; its attractiveness to oneself or other members of society. With yet more time, our nose may be relegated by evolution to just supporting the glasses on our face.

The nose also serves as a soundboard for emotional and sexual problems. The nasal membranes can react to anger, emotional excitement, and frustration. In such a reaction they can become blocked and discharge the watery mucus that presents itself in the common cold. Not only can an obstructed nose impair your breathing, but it could also interfere with your love life.

Variations on a Theme

Racial variations in nasal architecture are quite distinct and anthropologists use nose breadth and length as important measurements in racial classification. The warmer the climate, the wider its inhabitants' nostrils and the shorter their nasal bridges are apt to be, while those living in more glacial zones generally demonstrate a long, slender bridge and narrower nostrils. This allows the inhaled air to travel farther, absorbing warmth and moisture before entering the lungs. Thus the Nordic nose from an evolutionary standpoint is thin and high with narrow openings to the extreme cold. The nose of the African black is constructed for drawing large amounts of air from a humid, tropical climate.

Many cultures have focused attention on the nose. Primitive people thought that the kernel of life resided in the nostrils; thus they invested sneezing with a supernatural dread and significance. Certain South American Indians still seal the nose of the dead to prevent the person's ghost from escaping. Thrusting bones savagely through the nose, as ritualized by some African tribes, also is motivated by the idea of blocking death. More modern societies prefer superstitions such as associating itching of the nose with an approaching event or a right- or left-handed sneeze as favorable or unfavorable. We bestow a "Gesundheit" for a sneeze, not for a cough or hiccup. Although Western cultures view piercing the ears with rings as civilized, they regard nose rings with disfavor. A few cultures—notably the Eskimo and Polynesian—still respect the sexual aspect of the nose by substituting the rubbing of noses for the kissing ceremony.

Your Nose—The Long and Short of It

Countless books have been written on the intimate association between psychology and the nose. For as sensitive as the nose is to concussion, it is even more sensitive to criticism, real or imagined. One of the most regrettable of human peculiarities is the tendency to read personality traits in physical features. At one time schools of constitutional psychology actually emerged from the concept that appearance and personality are related. Examples include matching red hair with an explosive temper, thick lips with sensuality, and a high forehead with intelligence. The nose has its share of such stereotyping: we associate the hawk nose with cunning, the Roman nose with strength, the Greek nose with elegance and artistry, crooked noses with roughness and toughness, and on and on. Contemporary society has not yet reached a level of sophistication where it completely disregards such relationships among personality, character, and physiognomy. The human mind still assigns unpleasant qualities to an individual with unpleasant features.

In general, few people claim total contentment with the nose they were born with. Unlike other features, irregular, misshapen noses are the rule rather than the exception. In contrast to the mouth and eyes, the nose draws attention primarily when it is unattractive (large, melancholy eyes or beautifully sculptured lips may win compliments, but a well-shaped nose is usually unnoticed). As it stands out physically in any shape, it stands out even more when not consistent with the other features. Thus, the "perfect" nose is the one that fits the face behind it. And therefore, the object is not to make a perfect nose, but to construct a new nose harmonious with the face. Otherwise, one can perfect the nose, but ruin the face.

In addition to its prominence and central position, the nose is also the one major feature whose appearance is not readily improved with the application of cosmetics. However, it is one of the features that can be changed without outward evidence of surgery. These properties, plus the fact that nasal deformities are present in both sexes and at all ages, account for the great number of rhinoplasties performed; they tally at over 50 percent of all cosmetic operations.

Your Nose Can Get You in Trouble

The prominence and projection of the nose easily expose it to accidents first (and ridicule later—a case of adding insult to injury). Nasal fractures occur more often than to any other part of the human skeleton. In spite of this frequency, the treatment of nasal fractures lags behind that of similar traumas elsewhere in the body. While both physician and laymen realize that breaks of the extremities require immediate care, they seem unaware of the necessity for early corrective measures in fractures of the nose. Their casual attitude is based on the insignificant pain associated with nasal fractures (compared to that produced by such injuries elsewhere)—the small muscles surrounding the nose produce minimal muscle pull; therefore, the potential for pain is less. However, injuries are responsible for the great majority of nasal deviations.

The young in particular suffer from this lack of attention to "minor" nasal damage. Many physicians, in spite of their experience in other areas, cling to the peculiar theory that correction of posttraumatic nasal deformities should not be undertaken in children until their teens. This neglect can lead to functional and cosmetic abnormalities. The fractured bony fragments and twisted cartilage can obstruct the nasal passages, whose patency, or openness, is essential for proper respiration. The nasal sinuses can become infected and the obstruction can interfere with the sense of smell. Mouth breathing exposes the lungs to the damaging effects of cold, dry air that has not undergone warming, filtering, and humidifying via the nasal membranes. The open mouth also interferes with the normal forward and side movements of the tongue. The unopposed action of the facial muscles pressures the normal flat arch of the palate to develop a gothic shape which, in turn, produces dental distortion—crooked and otherwise irregular teeth, bad bite, and a small (weak) chin that imparts a languid expression to the face.

A deviated nose is a common deformity (Figure 2-1). Whatever

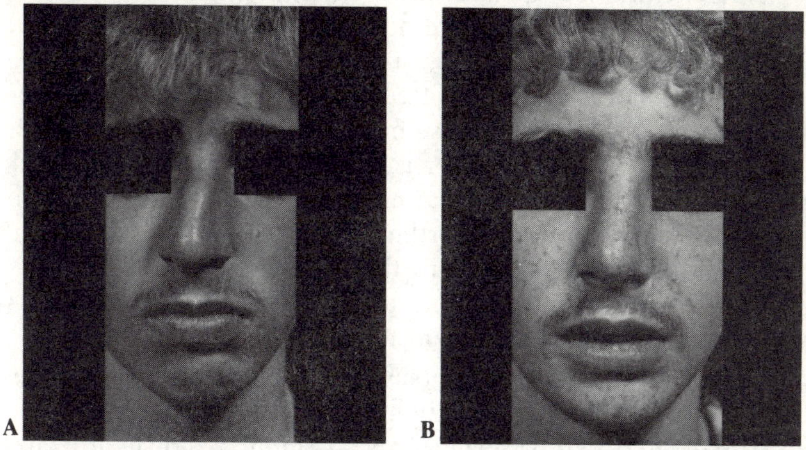

Figure 2-1 **A.** Teenager with marked deviation of bony and cartilaginous components causing manifest airway obstruction. **B.** Straightening the nose internally and externally allows normal nasal airflow—two weeks postoperative. (Same patient as in Figure 7-1.)

the external appearance, measures should be initiated to correct any internal cartilage which blocks the passage of air through the nose. With a blockage on one side of the nose, air cannot enter that side and absorb the moisture that is secreted by the membranes. This can lead to a postnasal drip or if the secretions pool and become stagnant, thickened yellow crusts will develop. With both sides blocked, not only do the above occur, but the continuous mouth breathing soon dries out the membranes of the throat, leaving it dry and irritable. And with one or both sides of the nose blocked, the person will usually snore (generally evidenced by conjugal protest).

The nose is responsible for our tossing and turning at night. Since we usually sleep on one side or the other, the lower nasal chamber closes off to rest while the upper one remains open to allow ingress of air. As the upper chamber fatigues, it slowly closes down and in so doing stimulates the neck to turn. This then transmits a neck reflex to the body, compelling it to twist in pursuit. The tired nasal chamber can now be allowed to rest while the refreshed chamber takes over the function of respiration.

As the Nose Grows

The nose, like the other facial features, continually changes as we mature. At birth and during early childhood, the nose has a flat shape and is tilted upward. Most external malformations, for example humps on the nose, are not usually evident until the initial growth periods have elapsed—about twelve or thirteen years for girls and fourteen or fifteen for boys. A bump, however, can appear at any age if the nose has been injured. Quite often the deformed nose of a teenager is secondary to an unrecognized fracture from childhood. It is during our adolescent years that we undergo the most rapid and startling emotional and physiological changes and it is also in the teens that an attractive self-appearance becomes most important. A bump can loom as big as a mountain during this adolescent turmoil.

The greatest number of rhinoplasties are performed during the late teens, as soon as the nasal bone growth is complete—approximately sixteen or seventeen years in girls and slightly later in boys. It is around this time, too, that the cartilaginous framework attains a degree of firmness. Removal of or incisions in the cartilage at an earlier age could result in a poorly shaped tip or nostril collapse since the immature cartilage does not mold well.

Growth of the nose ends with the late teens, but it continues to elongate throughout life from the constant pull of gravity. As we age, the appearance of the nose changes due to loss of skin elasticity, relaxation of the nasal muscles, and bone atrophy of the upper and lower jaws. The end result is a longer nose, curvature of the nasal bridge, and drooping of the tip. However, a nose that has undergone a rhinoplasty tends to resist elongation or dorsal curvature. This remarkable resistance to time and gravity is due to scar tissue formation that welds the overlying skin to the underlying tissues, stiffening the nasal structure against deforming forces.

Basically there is no age limit beyond which successful surgery cannot be performed. Although healing may be slower because of less nourishment to the structures, people in their fifties or sixties, if in good health, can undergo surgery without undue concern. The age limitation is physical rather than chronological. However, the older the individual, the less susceptible are the skin and tissue to remodeling and reshaping. This is caused primarily by the loss of skin elasticity whereby the skin may not drape as smoothly over the newly created framework.

Correcting a Flaw

The skin covering the nose has the same elasticity characteristic of skin elsewhere on the body and is quite capable of adjusting to substantial changes in the nasal framework wrought by the surgeon. Over the upper two-thirds of the nose, the skin feels loose and highly resilient; at the lower third it adheres more to the underlying structure and does not stretch as readily. Interiorly, the septum, a partition of bone and cartilage, divides the nose into two chambers. These nasal chambers, or cavities, are lined with tissue that warms, humidifies and filters inspired air and supplies the air conditioning requisite to proper respiration.

Certain types of nasal imperfections are more susceptible to correction than others. In general, a thin-skinned nose produces the most pleasing result. The sculpting of the underlying structures is displayed in vivid relief as the skin redrapes and hugs the revised frame, making the artistry of the surgeon vibrantly evident. Bony irregularities coupled with thin nasal skin promise classic improvement. Cartilaginous malformations are not so readily corrected and less satisfactory results are to be expected. Skin that is thick, oily, and replete with pores contracts poorly due to its restricted mobility and therefore cannot conform readily to the remodeled skeleton—its fit is loose like a chemise rather than tight like a knit. Incisions in such skin may heal with unnatural scarring and with a tendency toward irregularities of the underlying tissues. No matter what the designs created beneath the tissues, the thickened skin can mask precision surgery and thwart the finest artistic endeavors of the surgeon. Like sculptors, surgeons are also limited by the quality of their "marble."

The repair and artistic reshaping of the nose constitute one of the most exacting procedures in cosmetic surgery and if not respected as such, what is contracted to become a portrait can turn out to be a cartoon. The ability to ad lib during surgery may lend a virtuoso quality to rhinoplasty, but should never replace strategic thinking. The actual operative steps per se are reasonably easy, yet determining just how much to remove and how much to leave behind are what shapes the final outcome. The surgeon must not only study and visualize what is right for each patient, but he must also be capable of achieving this technically. When he decides on the height of the bridge, the character of the nose is established, and when he reconstructs the nasal tip, its attractiveness is gained or lost. Rhinoplasty is yet more exacting in that it comprises the sole cosmetic operation of the face where the surgical field is rigidly restricted. To correct a nose requiring only minimal improvement demands extreme precision and skill for more can be lost than gained within a precariously slim margin of tolerance—rhinoplasty has been correctly defined as the "surgery of millimeters." The craftsman must learn virtually to "see" with his fingertips, the feel of the newly created profile being equally if not more important than its visual impression. More often than not, a small defect in the new profile can be felt rather than seen.

Better Be Choosey

The interviews with the cosmetic surgeon are both physical and psychological. The surgeon gives physiological age more consideration than chronological age in deciding to operate. The operation should be discouraged in those with an unfavorable medical history unless the nasal physiology aggravates the problem. Without exaggeration we can state that the nose is the entrance to life and its normal physiology and critical air space should never be compromised to make its external appearance more attractive.

Psychological factors are probably the principal reason in rejecting a patient for rhinoplasty. Besides a nasal deformity, various motives can impel an individual to undergo surgery. These can range from marital difficulties, personal or business failures, feelings of depression and inferiority, to demands of a career in the public eye.

Some patients attempt to solve long-standing personality problems by instant anatomical changes. No amount of mere tinkering with appearances will solve the deeper problems of reality. A patient's undue concern over a minor nasal deformity could be the surface manifestation of a serious deep interpersonal problem. He may lose the physical scapegoat (his rationalization for failure) through surgery, but still may not be able to come to terms with himself emotionally. Psychologically disturbed people seldom show satisfaction with any cosmetic result. These patients, psychologically speaking, are in greater danger and deeper trouble than before because they no longer have any valid excuse for failure. It is not their nose that is out of sync; it is their psyche.

And as you might expect, there is a list of would-be patients who cannot understand why they are turned down by the surgeon: the person who wants all her features changed simultaneously with her nose; the individual who uses store mannikins as her models and wants her nose as flawless; the woman who requests a nose similar to that of some famous lady or reigning beauty queen; and those who come in carrying pictures of the nose they have picked out, although realistically it could not be achieved surgically with the tissues they possess.

In the following case history, a deep-rooted psychological disturbance underlying a deformed nose was uncovered following surgery. The case is interesting for entwined with the nasal appearance was a quiescent psychosis that was not picked up by the surgeon. Yet without the operation, the mental disorder might have erupted later in a much more violent and lethal fashion.

A thirty-year-old single Caucasian male requested a rhinoplasty. His nose, although quite wide at the bridge and projected somewhat high at the tip, was not unattractive. The patient, however, was visibly disturbed by it; in his words: "It spoils my looks" (which incidentally were rather nondescript).

After some consideration and since improvement was possible, the doctor agreed to perform the surgery. The nasal changes were discussed with the patient and he agreed with the surgical plan. The operation was performed, with the main efforts directed toward narrowing the bridge and reducing the tip height. The aesthetic change was subtle, but imparted a softer look to his face.

The patient, however, was unhappy; he stated that his appearance was not improved. Even when comparison was made with his preoperative photos, he refused to acknowlcdge that any change had occurred. In fact, he became extremely hostile when the pictures were displayed before him.

He was becoming very difficult to handle in the office when, late one evening, the situation climaxed in an emergency. The surgeon was summoned to a receiving hospital that had admitted the patient via a police ambulance. He had attacked and beaten his girl friend and subsequently had attempted suicide by barbiturate overdose.

The patient was comatose and in serious condition. The

woman, although swollen and bruised, was able to relate this story to the police and surgeon: her boyfriend was very angry and despondent over the outcome of his surgery. Nothing had changed for him. He had lost a promotion in an advertising agency to someone with less tenure (but more experience) and he blamed this on his appearance. She had also refused to continue seeing him because, although sometimes very charming, he was aloof and haughty in his manner and was both suspicious of and abrasive to all her friends. He blamed her refusal to continue seeing him on the belief that he was not "good looking enough for her." Yet she had told him that it was his personality, not his looks, that was ugly. He lamented to her that he felt as if he were slowly dying. And psychologically he was. Although he vented some anger on the surgeon, this was merely "window dressing," as he could not emotionally direct his full rage toward him.

Although the patient's convalescence was stormy, he recovered. The woman did not press charges. He was advised to stay away from her and ordered to seek psychiatric care, which he agreed to do. The therapy sessions uncovered an extremely unhappy childhood. He had been in numerous orphanages and foster homes since the age of four. His father had served time for fraud and as his mother worked, she could not care for him. At the age of eight, he returned to his parents; however, by then he had become an insecure child. As a youngster, he felt the reason he had been sent away from his parents was because he was bad, which he equated with being ugly. Whenever he failed at something (and he had a long history of having had many positions from which he had either been fired or had summarily left), he blamed it on his looks. Although his childhood had crippled him emotionally, in his mind's eye his face, and especially his nose, was the cause of his empty, desperate life.

He soon became aware that the only surgery he really needed was psychiatric. His negative and twisted personality was stripped to allow his rational being to emerge. He made several visits to the surgeon's office during these sessions, relating his progress. When finally discharged by the surgeon, he was well on his way to becoming a more secure and mature man; he was happier with himself and content with his nose.

People often complain of an inability to breathe via their nose or other functional disturbances in order to rationalize their need for surgery. Another interesting psychological aspect of rhinoplasty is that patients are often more critical about minor imperfections following surgery than about those wrought by nature. Small defects that would pass unnoticed in an unoperated nose may receive and attract comment out of proportion to their magnitude after a rhinoplasty. When the patient undergoes surgery, every flaw must be ironed out, a wish not always attainable.

The Surgical Strategy and Tactics

The operation itself is performed entirely within the nose with no visible scars resulting. The change in the nose structure is permanent. If the nostril width is reduced, a thin scar occurs within the base of the nose which in time fades and ultimately blends into the nostril border. Corrective nasal surgery consists of the following five steps: (1) elevating the skin from the bony and cartilaginous dorsum; (2) shortening the nose if necessary; (3) remodeling the tip of the nose; (4) removing the hump or lowering a prominent bridge to proportions consistent with the new tip; and (5) narrowing the nasal pyramid to compensate for the flatness caused by the hump removal. If indicated, this procedure can also be combined with the internal cartilaginous correction to improve the airway.

Removal of a nasal hump obligates the surgeon to break the nose (osteotomy), a surgical step that narrows the nose and is responsible for the majority of subsequent black-and-blue marks. The bridge of the nose outlines a pyramid, or roof gable, and removal of a hump simply truncates that pyramid or gable. The side walls must then be realigned to form the apex of the new pyramid at a lower level. If a hump is taken down without forming a new gable, the resulting flat-shaped nasal bridge is quite unattractive. Narrowing of the nasal bones also creates a visual effect of enlarged eyes by the imaginary widening of the space between them.

Management of the nasal tip probably constitutes the most exacting procedure of any rhinoplastic operation. Particularly in this region does the artistic judgment of the surgeon outweigh the purely technical aspects of surgery. It is the injudicious and/or unbalanced removal of the tip cartilages that usually produces the unsightly "operated look."

The shape of the tip is determined principally by the supporting cartilage. The appearance of the tip, however, may vary considerably from the basic cartilage structure, depending upon the skin thickness, underlying fat, and activity of the oil glands.

The angle the tip makes with the upper lip depends on its relative position with the neighboring fibrous attachments which suspend and stabilize it. Considerable change can be accomplished just by releasing the tip from the surrounding tissue. When the tip is elevated, the face appears more youthful and the upper lip appears wider, giving the person a more pleasant expression when laughing. Freeing the tip from its adjacent muscular attachment accounts for the temporary immobility of the upper lip and a change in the patient's smile. Within several weeks, however, muscle function returns as the tissues heal and the upper lip moves again in its usual fashion.

Variations among Races

The nasal deformities described up to now are distinctive for Caucasians. Non-Caucasians generally present a distinct set of nasal problems. Blacks and Orientals, when requesting surgery, desire a larger nose and higher bridge projection. Although the flat nose of the Black, with its low bridge and flaring nostrils may symbolize African beauty, the motivation for altering it can be just as complex as it is for Caucasians.

Rhinoplasty in black people generally involves raising the bridge, elevating the tip, and narrowing the width of the nostril floor. It is a more problematic undertaking than the usual caucasian nose as we must add rather than take away from the bridge, and incisions to narrow the nostrils tend to yield scars that can be more conspicuous in dark skin (Figure 2-2).

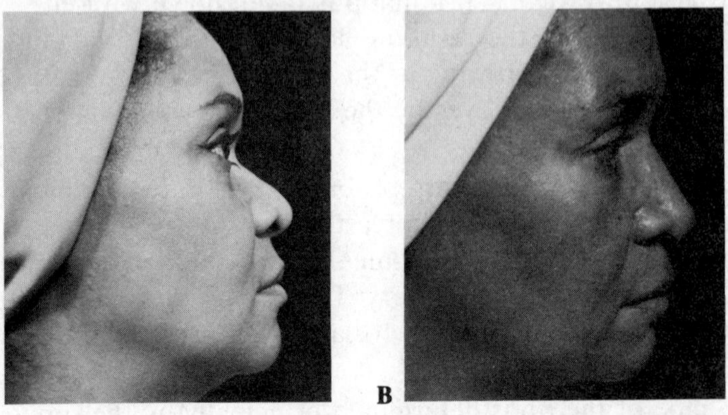

A B

Figure 2-2 A. There was a virtual absence of the nasal bridge producing an unattractive appearance. **B.** Dorsum augmented and nasal tip elevated using grafts from the septum—six months postoperative.

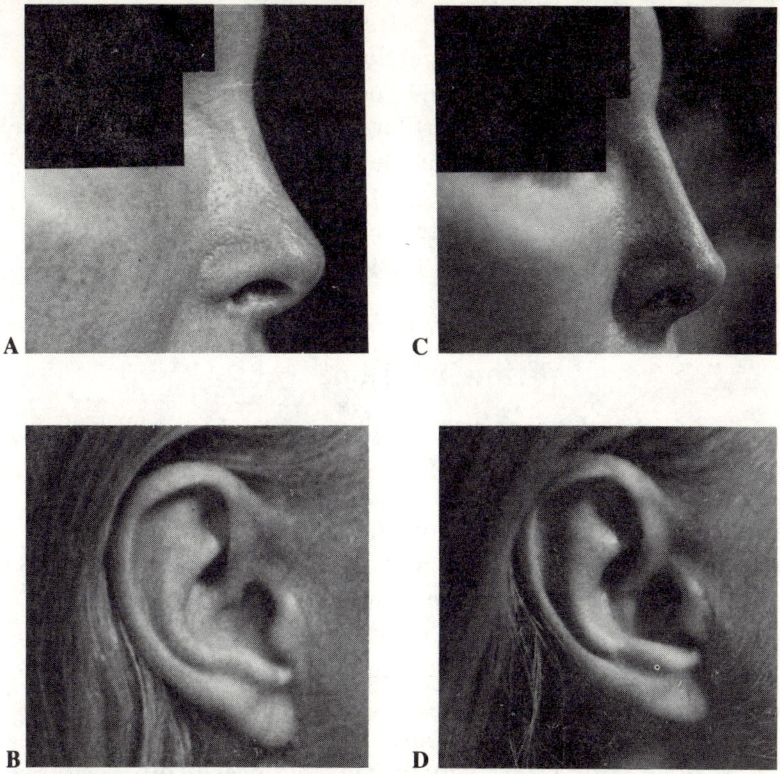

Figure 2-3 **A.** Patient had a retroussé and wanted a higher bridge; no septal tissue remained from previous surgery, therefore a cartilage graft from ear was used along the entire length of the bridge. **B.** Preoperative right ear. **C, D.** Addition of cartilage gives a stronger profile and more elegant look. No change in ear contour—two months postoperative.

Rhinoplasty is common among Orientals. It is a purely aesthetic procedure and ranks second in frequency to cosmetic surgery of the upper eyelid (in the Orient more reverence is given to the eyes than to the nose). The familiar triad of the flat nose, slant eyes, and prominent cheekbones produces the typical appearance of the Oriental. As in the black nose (and sometimes in Caucasians), cosmetic operations are essentially concerned with reshaping the nasal bridge by a graft or implant, associated with tip narrowing and remodeling. In the East, an implant rather than a graft is the substance predominantly used to augment the bridge.

A graft is living tissue separated from its original site

(occasionally from another person) and transferred to another region of the body; it is basically a transplant. A transplant is safer and offers less chance of infection than an implant, and should be used whenever feasible. The most readily obtainable and safest transplant to use is cartilage taken from the interior of the patient's nose. If this is not available, cartilage from the patient's ear can be used (Figure 2-3).* An implant is an inert substance buried beneath the skin and tissues of the body. Most implants used today are of some type of silicone. They are discussed more fully in chapter 7.

How It's Done

Prior to surgery, the patient enters the hospital for physical examination and routine laboratory tests. If the medical history suggests a tendency to bruise or bleed excessively, appropriate medication is administered approximately three to four days before surgery. Several hours before the operation, the patient is given pills and later, an injection to induce relaxation and a drowsy state. After being taken to the operating suite, the patient's face is cleansed and the face and body are draped with sterile sheets.

Most rhinoplasties are accomplished using a local analgesic, often in tandem with a light general anesthetic (which produces amnesia for the procedure). The nose is injected with the local analgesic agent. The heavy premedication together with the "twilight sleep" obliterates the needle pricks. All dissection is performed inside the nose. The surgeon slips a small scalpel between the skin and bone in each nasal chamber and frees the skin over the nasal architecture. Since the tip is met first it is the first part corrected. An incision within the nostrils exposes the cartilages that form the tip and nostril openings. These cartilages are dissected free and are trimmed to achieve the aesthetic result desired. Next the surgeon uses a small saw, rasp or chisel to remove the hump. This maneuver produces the truncated pyramid described above. Therefore, he introduces another chisel or saw to fracture the nasal bones and bring them toward the midline to form a new gable, or apex. The incision lines are stitched. The nose is packed internally to help mold it to its new

**Although the nasal bridge is composed of bone and cartilage, during surgery cartilage alone can be placed along the entire bridge to augment it. Under the skin, in this area, its appearance and feel are indistinguishable from bone.*

shape, and a plaster-of-paris splint dressing is applied to the outside to help retain the new shape and to protect the nose during the healing phase. The average rhinoplasty takes approximately one hour, depending on the experience and skill of the surgeon and the kind of nose presented.

This surgery, although not an involved operation, can be categorized as a major procedure. In the past, the operation was almost always performed in the hospital. This provided superior working conditions for the surgeon and allowed for more extensive remodeling as well as a greater margin of safety. With the inception of surgicenters and the furnishing of offices with modern surgical facilities, more and more rhinoplasties are being performed safely and competently as office procedures.

After the Break . . .

The mild discomfort that occurs after the operation stems mainly from the packing that is usually required to retain the changed structures in their new position. Since the patient is unable to breathe through the nose, mouth breathing makes the throat dry and irritated—the major complaints. Patients usually feel much better than they look at this stage, since bruising and swelling are very evident. Ice packs are often applied across the nose and eyes to diminish these common symptoms.

The patient stays in the hospital or office until sufficiently recovered from the anesthetic. Hospitalization can last from one to four days, depending upon the desires of the surgeon and patient.

The diet during the first few days is restricted to soft foods as excessive chewing can cause pain in the nasal tip and upper lip. When the packing and splint are removed on about the fourth or fifth day, the nose and eyelids will still be swollen. Strips of adhesive are then applied across the nose for the next few days. These help constrain the swelling, and more importantly, prevent the impression that what is present is the finished product. Within a week patients are usually presentable. In three weeks they are fairly well healed. Bruising generally disappears by the first week; the swelling lasts longer. The nasal skin, which initially is somewhat tense and shining, gradually returns to its normal texture. In some cases, this process can last for weeks or even months—after all, the nose is composed of many different tissues, each with a different healing potential and healing capacity. Thus, the success of a rhinoplasty should never be judged too soon after the operation as it may take months in some cases for the swelling to totally subside.

You can shampoo your hair one week after nasal surgery. If a hair dryer is used, it must be directed away from the nose. You can pluck your eyebrows in several days, but be careful to cleanse both the area and tweezers to prevent any infection. During the first week, mouth rinses or a water pick should replace teeth brushing. Barring that, brush your teeth gently. Cocktails are permissible several days after surgery, although they may cause your nose to swell more. For the first week, do not blow your nose; for several weeks thereafter only if necessary, and then gently with both nostrils open. Blowing the nose can trigger a nosebleed. Bleeding is a complication of rhinoplasty and when it occurs, the nose may require packing to stem the flow. This can prolong the convalescence and possibly alter the aesthetic result.

Long-Term Postoperative Care

The number of visits to the doctor's office afterward varies with the particular surgeon. Following removal of the nasal packing and splint, many surgeons observe the healing process weekly during the first month and once a month thereafter up to a year. Out-of-town patients should anticipate a week to ten days away from their homes. In these instances, long-term postoperative care is not practical (extended care, if needed, can be obtained from a physician closer to home).

Many factors can influence the healing after surgery. Sensitivity to drugs or even to adhesive tape can cause a nasal dermatitis resulting in redness and swelling of the nose which can inhibit healing. The patient's mental state can have a profound influence on healing. Psychologically composed patients heal more readily and with less care than those who are troubled. The surgeon can do much toward reassuring the patient, and this rapport must start with the initial consultation. The age of the patient also plays a great role in healing. The aged frequently recover slowly while the young demonstrate remarkable recuperative powers. Their bones, however, are not as easily fractured as are those of older individuals and thus, the osteotomy in the aged is rarely a challenge. The nutritional status of the patient is also important; patients deficient in protein heal more slowly and are more prone to infection than those in a good nutritional state.

After the nose has completely healed, it requires no special precautions. However, during the immediate postoperative period, many activities must be curtailed. It is in this crucial period that the cosmetic result achieved by the surgeon is susceptible to damage by the patient's casual behavior. Only after the splint and subsequent tapes have been removed should one shower. Until then, the patient may take a bath, being careful to prevent slipping or submerging the head. Smoking should also be avoided for the first few weeks (the nose has been irritated enough without adding smoke to the membranes). Air travel should be postponed for one week following surgery (although planes are pressurized, a possible pressure differential upon landing could start a nosebleed in the still-healing vessels).

Sunbathing should be avoided for approximately one and a half months; excessive heat and ultraviolet radiation will cause swelling, peeling, and irritation of the nasal skin. Patients who wear eyeglasses must be cautious for six weeks—their pressure

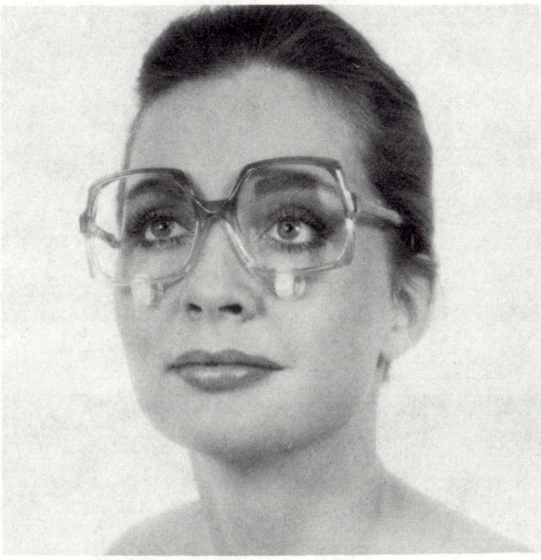

Figure 2-4 All pressure from glasses transferred to cheeks thus avoiding the possible formation of pressure dents.

creates redness and depressions on the side of the nose. If they are absolutely necessary, they can be suspended from the forehead with cellophane tape or fitted with Frame-ups*. These transparent clip pads allow the glasses to rest on the cheeks rather than on the nose (Figure 2-4).

**Obtainable from Arox Co., P.O. Box 24740, Los Angeles, CA 90024 ($3).*

Depending on the social and physical aspects of their occupation, patients can usually return to work or school in about one week. However, they should shun strenuous sports, such as swimming, tennis, and handball for six weeks. Walking is permissible the next day; jogging after two weeks. For several weeks, sexual activities should exclude the head and neck. "Necking," in particular, frequently injures the nose.

The patient should not touch his nose for several weeks following surgery. Cleansing of the face at this time should exclude the nose. On occasion, there are patients with wide nasal bones or those whose nasal bones have a tendency to spread apart. In these cases, a simple manual exercise will aid in the retention of the new shape. It consists of a twice-daily five-minute

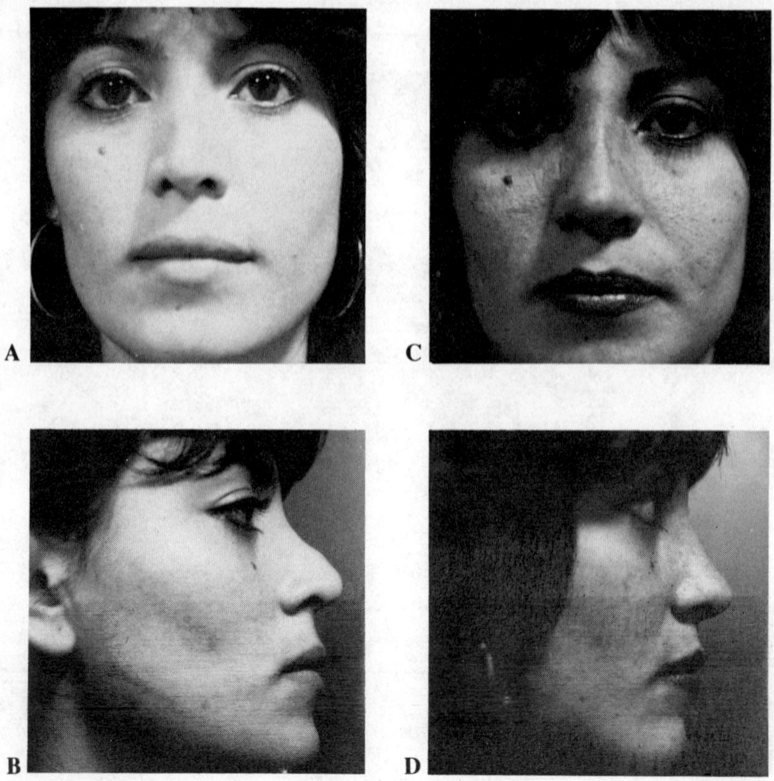

Figure 2-5 A, B. Young patient had excessive bone and inadequate cartilage removed with previous rhinoplasty. **C, D.** Excess cartilage from behind the tip removed, fashioned and placed higher along the bridge. Note how much more the eyes stand out after the bridge is built up—seven months postoperative.

stint wherein the forefingers, placed along and parallel to the bones, exert pressure downward and inward. Within a relatively short time, the nasal bones will retain their position, and remain stationary.

Ideally the nose should be reshaped with the least possible indication that a surgeon has tampered with it. Contrary to the common assertion that a rhinoplasty can be easily spotted, when properly performed, not even the most experienced cosmetic surgeon can detect an operated nose without internal examination. However, approximately 5 to 10 percent of all rhinoplastic operations do not turn out as desired because of excess scar tissue formation, injury during the healing phase, or other untoward developments. The operation can be repeated successfully if sufficient cartilage and bone are left from the previous surgery (Figure 2-5). Even without adequate remaining tissue, grafts or implants can be used to further embellish the nose. However, with each successive operation, scar tissue, unlike normal tissue, may heal and contract in an unpredictable manner. The chances of success, even though adequate tissue remains, decrease with each surgical procedure and the artistic result is likely to be less than perfect.

The Price Is Right!

The surgical fee varies from surgeon to surgeon. It is determined by his experience, his reputation, the area of the country in which he practices, and the type of nose that he must correct. On the average, the charge for a rhinoplasty is not less than $2500; higher fees are not uncommon. Septal (cartilage) surgery is an integral part of rhinoplasty; therefore, whether performed at the office or in the hospital, the procedure and hospitalization are always defrayed by insurance.

Whatever the cost, the price is worth it for facial improvement obtained through rhinoplasty can come close to magic. The following history is illustrative: Janet, a seventeen-year-old high school senior, was in many ways a model youngster. Her grades were good, she was a voracious reader and enjoyed pondering philosophical issues. There were no apparent family squabbles or sibling rivalries. Her parents, however, were concerned with her reclusive behavior for she was constantly at home neither attending parties nor going out with boys. It was her parents who had urged her to come into the office. She had a large nose which she had always, lightheartedly, referred to as her "hook," but they suspected that her looks bothered her more than she would ever confide in them.

Her face, which was more honest than pretty, was overwhelmed by a very large nose that obscured her large eyes and flawless complexion. As the discussion became more comfortable for her, her shyness dissolved like a fog and in a babbling manner she admitted that she had never, ever felt pretty. Since she thought that boys could see better than they could think, she was afraid that her awkward looks would be a turn-off, as had actually happened many times in her early teens. She had turned inward to books and herself for refuge and security. "I don't want to be beautiful;" "I've never been beautiful;" "I would just like to look nice."

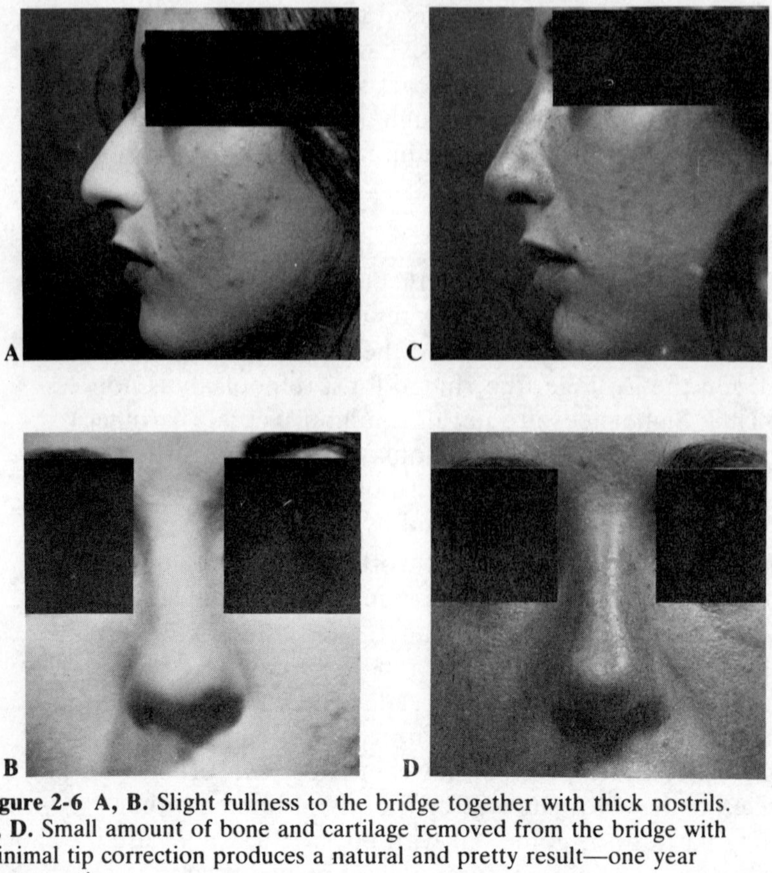

Figure 2-6 A, B. Slight fullness to the bridge together with thick nostrils. **C, D.** Small amount of bone and cartilage removed from the bridge with minimal tip correction produces a natural and pretty result—one year postoperative.

The doctor discussed the surgical changes with her and her parents. The surgery was uneventful. On the day of the unveiling, she was excited, even trembling. As she looked at her new nose, it was like watching a butterfly emerge from a cocoon. She turned to the surgeon and said: "Oh, doctor, it's such a pleasure to look good." And "look good" was an understatement. The lowering of her bridge and narrowing of the tip had transformed her into a beauty. As she continued to gaze at her reflection, one could see that at last, her archenemy, the mirror, had finally become her friend.

The Moment of Truth

The dramatic unveiling of the nose, when the splint is removed, is a momentous event in the patient's life. It can be a moment of

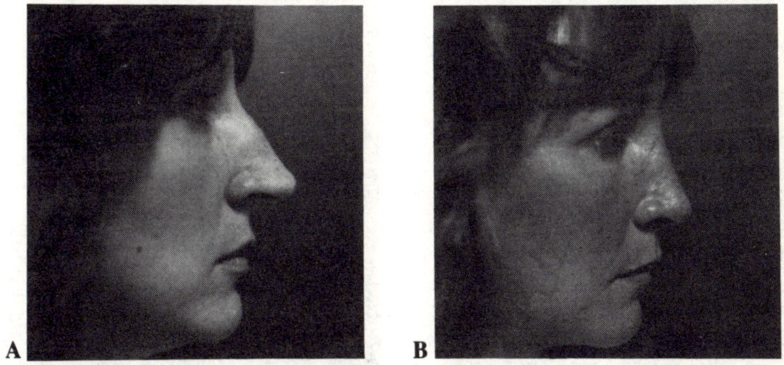

Figure 2-7 A. Large nose with moderate hump and long, projecting tip. **B.** Minimal hump removed, but extensive tip remodeling with dramatic result—two years postoperative.

great exhilaration. A long-awaited dream for a new and more attractive appearance is about to come true. Despite the swelling, despite the bruising, the effect is moving. At long last, the patient experiences a sense of his or her own beauty. As patients acclimate to this new awareness of their own attractiveness, feelings of inadequacy disappear along with the fear of meeting people. There is a new confidence and greater self-esteem. With the deformity dissolved under the surgeon's scalpel, the impeding neuroses seemingly evaporate. The death of the old deformity gives birth to a new personality (Figures 2-6, 7, 8, 9).

Anyone in serious doubt of the remarkable benefits of

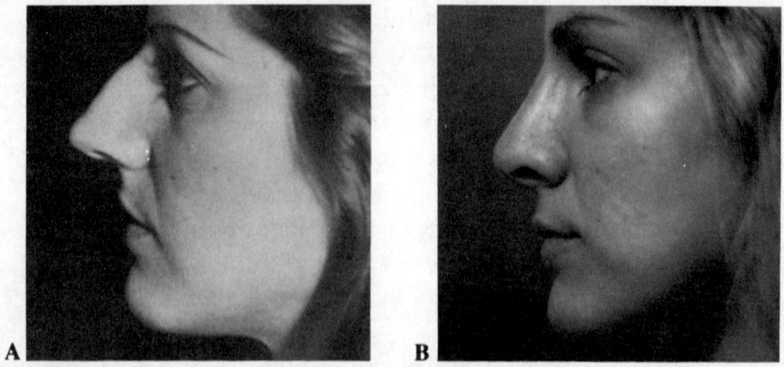

Figure 2-8 A. Large, misshapen nose throwing entire face out of balance. **B.** Major reduction of all components producing a harmonious, pleasant result—one year postoperative.

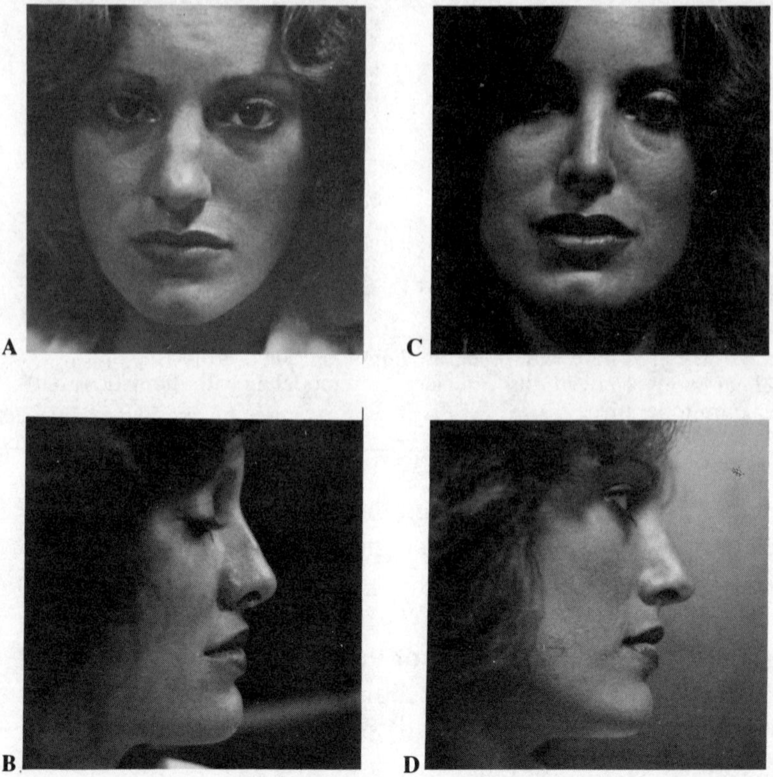

Figure 2-9 A, B. Young model whose flawless face was marred by wide, irregular nasal bones. **C, D.** Subtle refinement of bridge and narrowing of nasal bones yields a more photogenic look—one year postoperative.

rhinoplasty need only talk to a person who has had a successful operation. Perhaps the most compelling measure of the breadth and pace and growth of rhinoplastic surgery is the acceptance that people have given it; without question, it is the most frequently requested cosmetic operation and it is a reasonably safe bet that this popularity will continue. As imaginative approaches to correct the unattractive or deformed nose are continually being developed, by the turn of the century the cosmetic surgeon will undoubtedly have a new twist on how to straighten a crooked nose.

Q&A

Is it necessary to break my nose?

Rhinoplasty almost always embraces restructuring of the entire nose. Thus, removing the hump requires breaking the nose to reform and narrow the bridge. When only the tip is deformed (rare) or a rhinoplasty has miscarried leaving the tip unnatural-looking, an isolated tip procedure can be performed without disturbing the bridge.

How long will I need to wear a bandage over my nose?

Approximately seven days: four to five days for the plaster-of-paris splint to maintain the new position of the fractured bones and several days of tape thereafter to inhibit the soft-tissue swelling that occurs.

Will it interfere with my breathing?

At first, yes. Remember the nose has been cosmetically injured and there is just as much swelling occurring on the inside as there is on the outside. As the swelling subsides (several weeks and in some cases, months), nasal breathing will return to normal. This discomfort is the predominant complaint as, for the majority of patients, there is virtually no pain following this procedure.

When is the best age to have a rhinoplasty?

After nasal growth is finished, approximately sixteen years in females and eighteen years in males. Extenuating circumstances could warrant nasal surgery at an earlier age; however, classic results generally occur when the nose is operated upon after that feature has reached full growth.

Why is the surgery expensive?

More often than not the surgeon must create harmony out of disharmony and order out of chaos. The surgical artistry is so involved and the skill so instinctive that it borders on genius. You are paying for that remarkable talent and the price is generally high.

3

The Eyelids—There's More Than Meets the Eye

Philosophers and poets have called eyes the mirrors of the soul. Unfortunately, these mirrors can reflect a portrait of old age more vividly than any other facial feature. The eyes and nose compete for attention, but unlike the nose, the expressive action of the eyes magnifies even the slightest blemish. And for the most part, it is imperfections about the lids which impart an aged and tired look to the face.

The unattractiveness of wrinkles and bags, skin folds, and sags can be improved with an "eye-lift," also known in cosmetic surgery as a blepharoplasty. The operation achieves a smoothing out of wrinkles and under-eye bags, a lifting of drooping lids and brows and, if need be, a reshaping of the eyelid by changing its size or slant. Blepharoplasty is the second most common operation performed by the cosmetic surgeon.

Bulges, Bags, and Fat

The skin of the upper eyelid is the thinnest in the body. It folds readily, allowing rapid opening and closing of the eye. This thinness also induces early wrinkling. Except along the lid margin, the skin is loosely connected to the underlying tissue and can swell easily. Any injury to that area or allergic phenomenon produces an immediate display of the skin's increased volume. When the eye opens, the loose skin of the upper lid forms several horizontal folds; in particular, one well-marked fold can be seen along the upper frame of the lid.

During the aging process, the skin undergoes thinning and loss of elasticity, and the tone of the underlying muscles and tissues diminishes (see chapter 5). As these changes evolve, the skin lines formed by action of the eyelid muscles develop into deeper and more permanent creases. Wrinkles form across the lower lids and others fan outward from the eye. Women are unable to apply makeup securely as opening and closing the eye smears powder and eyeliner in the accordionlike creases. Herniation of the deep eye fat, which bulges out between the eye muscles, produces a generalized pouch in the lower lids. In the upper lids a skin redundancy occurs, forming a hood to the eye. Herniation of orbital fat into the lid also occurs, together with a drooping of the eyebrow.

Eyelid wrinkles usually develop around the twenty-fifth year and imprint more deeply with age. Lower-lid bags also emerge early in life, depending on genetic inheritance, allergies, and living style. With age, the upper lid progressively lowers to the extent that, in some cases, it can block the vision, particularly in upper and outer gaze. The sagging, heavy upper lid requires more energy to raise it and therefore the eyes tire easily. The drooping lids can also cause headaches in some people as a result of the excess burden placed on the forehead muscles in their attempt to help raise the lids.

A drooping brow can also contribute to sagging of the upper lid. Correction of the brow not only returns it to a more youthful position but, as a bonus, also softens the crow's feet and occasionally even eliminates them.

The origin of eyelid bags is still a medical uncertainty. While a number of diseases are responsible in some cases, no direct cause has been determined. Dissipation or merely excesses in living are often cited. Subjecting the body to unrelenting stress can produce the bags; however, genetic traits contribute significantly. Because the baggy-eyed person is often accused of dissipation or thought to be unhealthy, he may suffer psychologically more from this indictment than from the problem of the deformity itself. When it comes to looks or morals, one is rarely given the benefit of the doubt.

Development of eyelid bags is intimately associated with herniated orbital fat. Deep orbital fat forms a soft cushion behind the eyeball and serves as a shock absorber for the eye. These fat cells do not respond to dieting and remain even if the body becomes extremely emaciated. You cannot get rid of herniated fat by lowering your food intake.

Normally, the eye muscles and deep fibers prevent the fat from spilling out into the lids. As the muscles and tissue weaken, however, the fatty structure bulges forward against the muscle and skin. Although these pockets are known as herniated orbital fat, the condition is not comparable to other hernias of the body such as in the groin or abdomen. That is, it is not associated with a breach in a single orifice or the straining of tissue. The protrusion cannot be corrected by placing the fat back into its proper position, followed by tightening or strengthening the surrounding tissue; it must be removed. Herniation may precede wrinkling and excess skin; however, the bulging fat eventually causes enough stretching to produce the pouches, or bags. The condition may be present in both upper and lower lids, but it is more visible in the lower lid and cosmetically more disturbing (Figure 3–1).

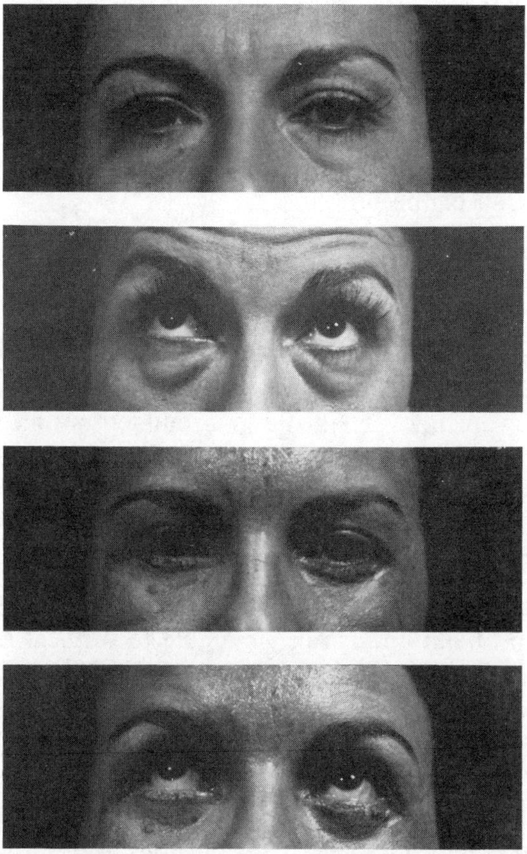

A B C D

Figure 3-1 A, B. Herniated fat in the lower lid creating an aged, tired appearance. **C, D.** Five days postoperative. There are several sutures remaining in the outer incision area. Despite some swelling and crusting along the lid incision, a more youthful look is already manifest.

Meet Leticia

Leticia was in her mid-twenties when she consulted me about a blepharoplasty. From childhood through her teens she had suffered from hay fever and had undergone the ritual tests and therapy to alleviate her symptoms. She had also suffered a severe attack of tonsillitis as a child and the infection had spread to her kidneys, causing damage to one of them. Both her kidney and allergic problems continued to plague her during her early years.

From the first time that she could recall looking into a mirror, she noted that her eyes were always puffy. This was attributed to either her allergies or her chronic kidney condition. As she matured, her allergies became more quiescent and her renal flare-ups less frequent; however, she still retained a constant puffiness in the upper and lower lids. In her twenties, a detailed study by her physicians revealed that her puffiness was not caused by any disease or allergic process, but by herniated fat which swelled from her body fluids. Because the appearance was so disturbing to her, she elected to undergo surgical removal of the herniated fat and rid herself of the problem.

Examination revealed fullness in both upper and lower lids. Since the fat acted like a sponge and retained fluid, she was given a diuretic and placed on a salt-free diet several days before surgery. Ridding the fat of excess fluid would give the surgeon a clearer picture of how much fat to remove. The surgery and convalescence were uneventful. Leticia retained her allergies and intermittent kidney problem; she lost the puffiness around her eyes.

Shiners

Discoloration beneath the lids is a vascular (blood vessel) or pigmentation problem and is not amenable to surgical relief. The condition is often referred to as "allergic shiners," as it arises in those with a long-standing history of nasal allergies. With severe nasal congestion, the normal circulatory flow about the lower lids is obstructed, causing the veins to engorge and bulge, which can be seen through the skin. (The dark shadows and circles beneath the lids are similar to the black eyes that follow an injury—thus the designation.) This engorgement also produces swelling which can be misinterpreted as herniated fat. Treatment is directed toward clearing of the nasal congestion through appropriate anti-allergic medication. As this condition is common among children, early measures should be instituted to prevent its continuance into adult life.

Injuries and insect bites frequently cause temporary damage to the lids. Because of the loose attachment of the underlying tissues, blood and serum easily seep through the tissues causing rapid swelling and bruising. The black eye is predominantly a cosmetic problem and is usually absorbed within one to two weeks. The immediate application of direct pressure and cold compresses over the lid following injury can suppress some of the swelling and bruising. In the past, doctors placed leeches over the black-and-blue areas to draw out the blood. In present-day society, using blood-suckers on the face is not the "in" thing to do.*

How It's Done

Basically, the eyelid operation consists of making an incision in the fold of the upper eyelid and removing the excess skin and fat. With a comparable incision below the lash line on the lower lid, the surgeon can elevate the skin, reach in and remove the protruding fat, and cut away the excess skin to give a smoother look. Dynamic lines—those formed by smiling and laughing—although improved, cannot be removed completely by this operation. It is the unwanted skin, wrinkles, and pouches present in a static pose that are within the purview of this surgery and it is these flaws that can be dramatically improved with blepharoplasty.

The surgery is performed either under a local or general anesthetic and as an office or hospital procedure. The patient is handled in the usual fashion preoperatively (sedation, prepping, draping, and so on) and while he or she is in the upright position, the incision lines are outlined with a marking pen (Figure 3-2). In this manner, the surgeon can determine more accurately the amount of skin that can be excised safely from the lids. When the patient is placed in the supine position, the local analgesic is administered and the sculpting begins.

From a surgical standpoint, separate operations for the upper and lower lids are ideal; however, many patients cannot afford the extra time off for the two surgeries. Therefore, the two lid

**Another reason one may not want leeches is because once they become attached and bloated with blood, they are difficult to remove. They must be burned off (a cigarette is the best way). If pulled away, a part of the head can remain lodged within the tissues and promote an infection.*

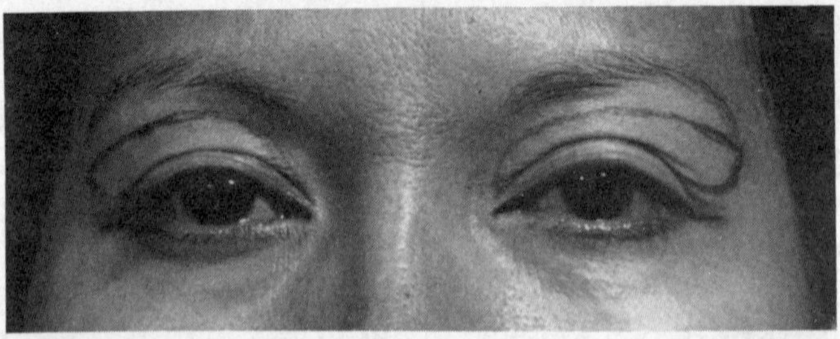

A

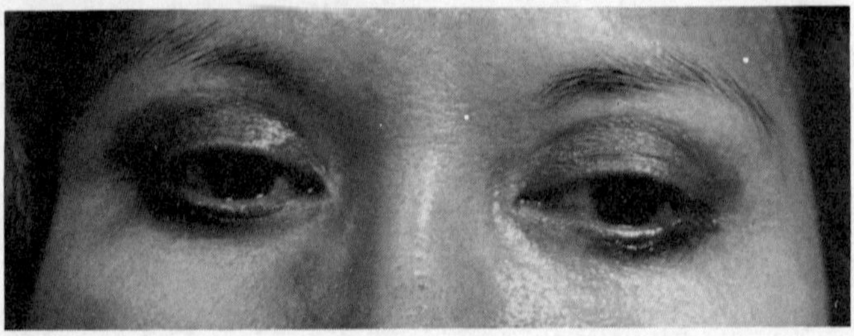

B

Figure 3-2 **A.** Incisions outlined in gentian violet. **B.** Two months postoperative.

procedures are generally combined into a single session. The sequence of the lid operations varies with each surgeon; many prefer to operate on the lower lids first, as they require greater detail, precision, and skill.

The incision in the lower lid carries slightly lateral from the inner corner of the eye into a crease line immediately below the lid, parallels that lid to the outer corner of the eye, and then slopes into a laugh line for a distance of four to five millimeters. The surgeon then frees the lower lid skin from the underlying tissues and exposes the bulging fat. This is removed to leave a smooth surface in place of the bulges. The skin is then draped in an upward and lateral direction and the excess cut away. The surgeon closes the incision using fine sutures. The resultant thin scar is easily masked beneath the lashes and by the outer smile line.

There is another approach for lower lid bags. The surgeon pulls the lid away from the eye and makes a horizontal incision across the pink tissue within the lid. Through this internal incision, he can remove the bulging fat without leaving any tell-tale evidence of a scar. However, with this method, no skin slack can be removed; therefore, it is reserved for young patients with only fat protrusion and no excess skin.

The surgeon corrects the upper lid by removing the previously outlined segment of skin and by removing the excess fat within the upper lid. He closes the incision with the same suture material used for the lower lid. The scar, nestling in the normal furrow of the upper lid, is completely hidden. Sterile ice packs are draped over the eye and the lid procedures are repeated on the opposite side.At the completion of the surgery, the lids of both eyes are covered with gauze, and ice packs are reapplied to inhibit the bruising and swelling. As much as possible, ice will be applied to the eyes for the remainder of the day. The surgical time for the repair of the upper and lower lids is approximately two hours; for the lower lids alone, one-and-one-half hours are required; for the upper lids, about thirty minutes.

If there is a deep frown present, this can be softened when the upper lid is corrected. At the inner aspect of the upper lid incision, the surgeon introduces a fine scissors just beneath the skin and spreads it upwards toward the frown. He then severs the skin from the underlying muscle. Portions of fat removed from the lids can be introduced into this area to fill out the frown (Figure 3-3). Occasionally, just the separation that releases the

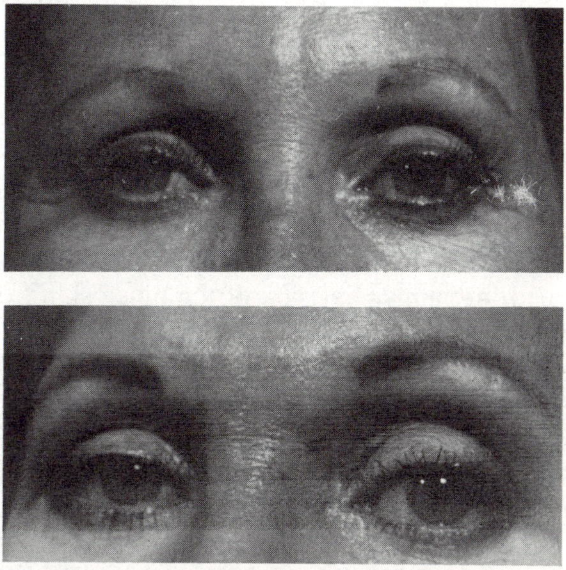

A

B

Figure 3-3 A. Deep, glabellar depression imparting a continuous frown. **B.** Frown improved by insertion of fat through minute stab incision within the left upper lid area—four weeks postoperative.

frown from the muscle will stimulate the production of scar tissue beneath the skin, thereby creating a softening effect. The same result can also be accomplished via a stab approach through the eyebrow if no upper lid procedure is contemplated. Thus, like the methods mentioned in chapter 4, these procedures can also be used without leaving any visible scar.

Correction of drooping eyebrows is accomplished by removing an ellipse of forehead skin just above and lateral to the brow. The amount of skin resected depends on the amount of elevation required to restore the brows to a more youthful level. Most of the resultant scar is hidden in the brow; the rest, which is more exposed, requires make-up for camouflage. When necessary, the brow lift can be performed in conjunction with upper and lower lid blepharoplasties.

Careful As We Go

Blepharoplasty comprises one of the most delicate and precise cosmetic operations. Although many features can be and are altered at one sitting, the fatigue of both surgeon and patient in a lengthy session, together with the increased bruising and swelling that can occur, may yield results that are often less than desired. Eyelid repair is best carried out as an isolated surgery, for it is an exacting procedure and tolerates only a slim margin of error; it should not be performed with a face-lift. These two surgeries produce the best results when performed at least one day apart, with the lids being repaired first.

Because the operation is bilateral, symmetry must be achieved between the eyes. Minor differences between the two will draw more attention than a black eye. Taking out too much fat replaces a bulge with a hollow, a maneuver guaranteed to leave the patient far from happy. Excision of too much skin from the lower lid will leave a too-taut lid that will pull the eyelid down, giving a "hound-dog" appearance and causing the eye to water. Removing too much skin from the upper lid will interfere with natural closure of that lid, producing a dry and painful eye, possible infection, and visual disturbances. Any attempt to remove every wrinkle in the lids to obtain a "manicured" look is extremely hazardous. The risks are real and can be catastrophic when they occur. The surgeon's main endeavor is to clear up the eyelid expression and produce more youthful-looking eyes.

If any noticeable wrinkles persist that disturb the patient, lid chemosurgery can be performed approximately two months after surgery. As a rule, this will ameliorate them (see chapter 5).

Eyeing the Results

Eyelid sutures are usually removed by the third or fourth day following surgery. Brow sutures are left for approximately seven days. The patient may wear sunglasses by the second postoperative day, and can insert contact lenses within five or six days. Reading and watching TV are possible by the second or third day.* Hair may be shampooed on the third postoperative day; any sutures still remaining will not become a problem if they become damp. After the second week, patients may wear full eye makeup. They can usually return to work within seven to ten days when both the upper and lower lids are corrected; within three to five days when just the uppers are repaired; and within one week when only the lowers are corrected. In each case, there may be some swelling and bruising, but these can be concealed with sunglasses or makeup.

The incisions will remain pink for several months, but make-up will mask these. Two or three months following the surgery, the scars, in most cases, will fade and blend with the normal skin

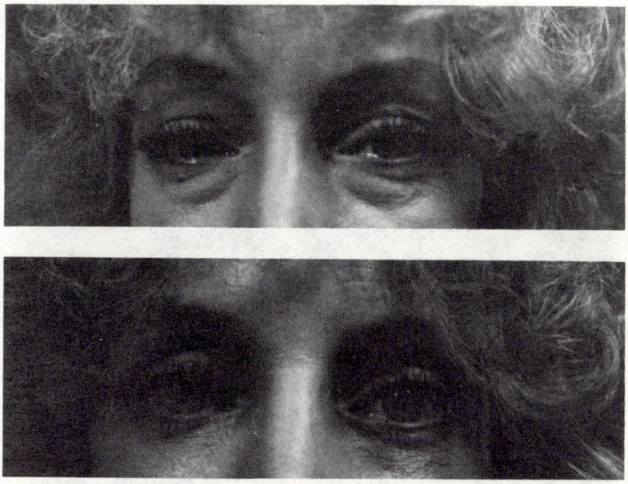

A

B

Figure 3-4 A. Herniated fat in all compartments of upper and lower lids. **B.** Six months postoperative.

**The vision may be blurred due to the swelling and eye watering that may occur. However, this is temporary and the visual acuity will return to normal within several days.*

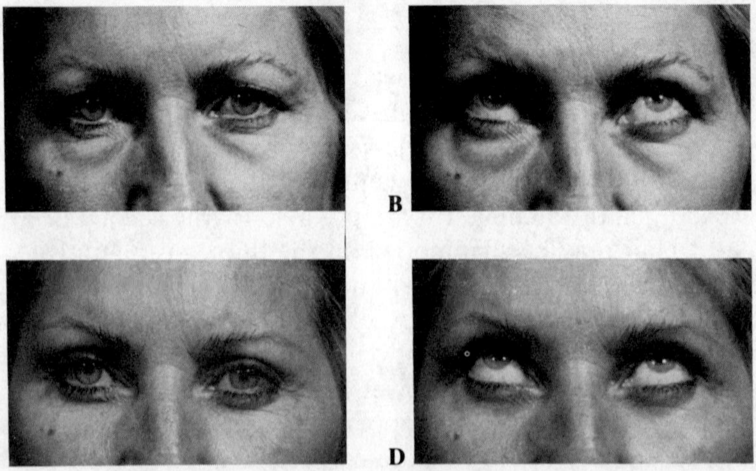

A B C D

Figure 3-5 A, B. Herniated fat in all compartments with minimal excess skin. **C, D.** Fat removed with rotation of skin upward and laterally. Only lateral skin excess requires removal to produce a smooth, taut lower lid—eight months postoperative.

lines of the lids. The thin skin of the lids heals with virtually invisible remnants of the cut. The scar along the eyebrows requires more time to fade. It may not be as fine and can be difficult to conceal.

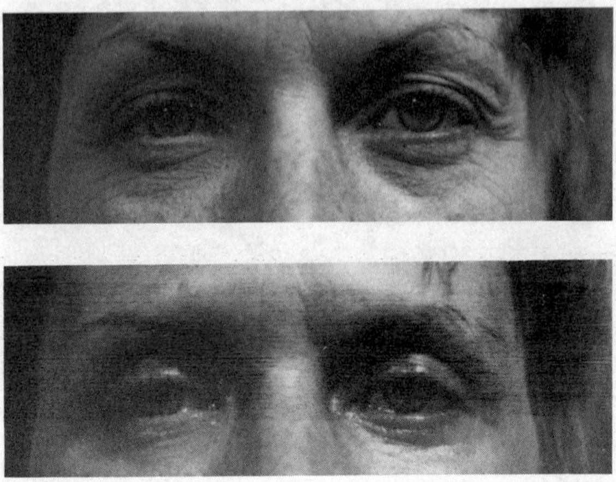

A B

Figure 3-6 A. Excess skin in upper and lower lids. **B.** Upper and lower blepharoplasty mainly removing redundant skin and minimal fat excision—two weeks postoperatively.

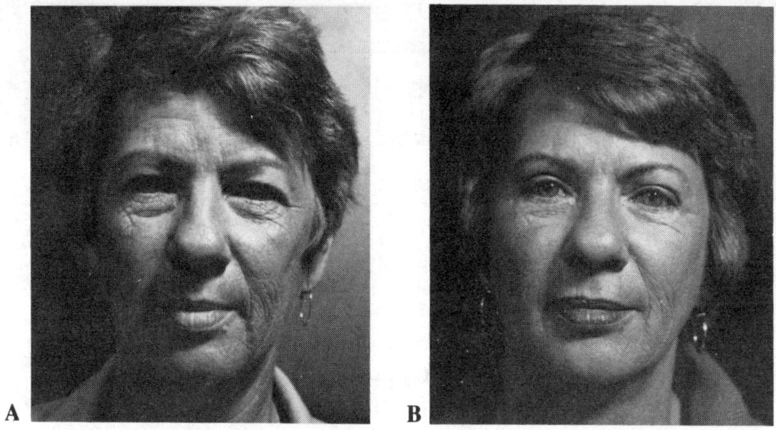

Figure 3-7 A. Weather-beaten skin and marked sagging and wrinkling of eyelids. **B.** Five months postoperative. Upper and lower lid repair improves the appearance of the eyes. A later peel puts frosting on the cake; see chapter 5.

How long a blepharoplasty will last varies with each patient and particularly with the individual's style of living. Because the upper third of the face stretches and sags less with aging than the lower two-thirds, eyelid and brow corrections are more durable than face-lifts. The patient will continue to age, but the upper and lower lid skin will be smoother and tighter than it would have been without surgery. Some examples of blepharoplasty are

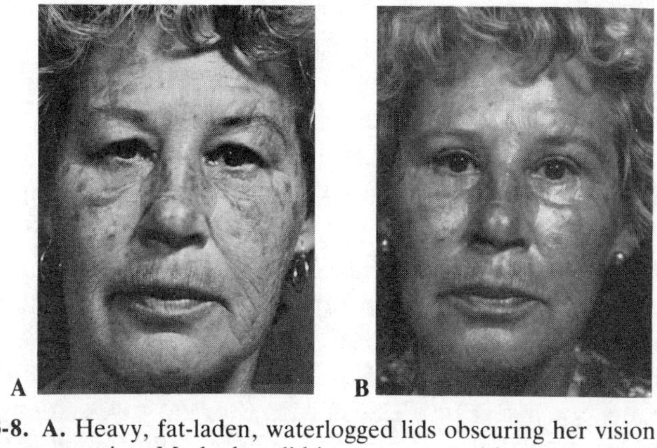

Figure 3-8. A. Heavy, fat-laden, waterlogged lids obscuring her vision. **B.** Eight months postoperative. Marked eyelid improvement with surgery. Face peeling yields an added dividend; see chapter 5.

illustrated in Figures 3-4, 5, 6, 7, 8.

After the eyelids are repaired, the patient can prevent puffiness that occurs upon arising in the morning by placing a one and a half inch block of wood under each leg at the head of the bed. During sleep, the orthostatic (straight-standing) fluid pressure then flows toward the feet (as it does when standing all day) and your lids will no longer have that early morning swollen appearance.

The Oriental Eye

Within the domain of blepharoplasty is the oriental eye procedure, a type of surgery that departs slightly from the conventional operation. Some Occidentals want their eyes converted to an oriental cast, or "doe" look; Orientals wish their eyelids changed to a Western eye. The latter surgery has increased enormously among Asians as the American influence has spread throughout the Orient. Remodeling the oriental eye to occidental form is a simple twenty-minute operation in the Orient, and by far the most widespread cosmetic operation in that region of the world.

There are distinctive anatomic variations that distinguish the mongoloid from the occidental upper lid. The oriental eye lacks the palpebral fold (or furrow) found in the Westerner's upper lid; hence, there is no "double eye" fold and the lid, which also contains a surplus of fat, hangs down like a drooping curtain, concealing part of the colored portion of the eye. This produces an image that has unfortunately been associated with mystery, inscrutability, and the arcane. In addition, the outer corner of the oriental eye tends to be somewhat higher than the inner, giving the eye an upward slant. And in about 50 percent of Orientals, a fold of skin (the epicanthal fold) curves down toward the nose and obscures the inner corner of the eye.

The oriental-to-occidental lid procedure differs slightly from the usual upper blepharoplasty. In these cases, a fold must be created where none existed. After the surgeon has excised the required amount of skin from the lid and removed the fat, he identifies the muscle expansion (the end fibers) that raises the lid and sews this expansion to the remaining skin (in the Oriental, these muscle end fibers do not insert into the skin as they do in Occidentals). When the eye opens, the eyelid skin is now pulled upward and backward, thereby giving rise to the palpebral fold. The fibrous tissue formation that develops at these sites perpetuates the fold.

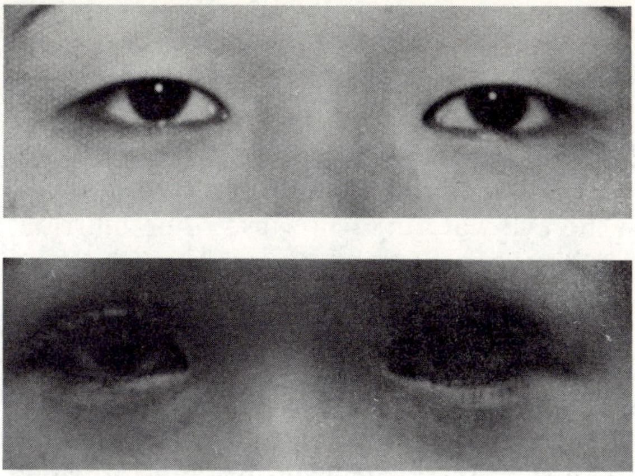

Figure 3-9 **A.** Typical, full upper lid of oriental. **B.** Superior palpebral cleft now evident after surgery—three months postoperative.

The incision is closed in the usual fashion and the postoperative care is the same as for the conventional blepharoplasty (Figure 3-9). (If the epicanthal fold is to be corrected, it is done via a "Z" plasty, which is the exchange of two triangular skin flaps.)

Looking at the Cost

Fees for conventional upper and lower blepharoplasty vary between $2000 and $2500. Upper or lower blepharoplasty alone entails an expense of from $1000 to $1500. The cost of westernizing the oriental lid ranges from $1000 to $1500, as does a brow-lift. If it can be shown by photographs and proven by visual tests that the upper-lid sag interfered with vision, the patient's insurance will defray part of the surgical cost. Lid surgeries as a rule are not covered by insurance.

The stimulus for this surgery is the desire for a more youthful appearance because imperfections of the lids, unlike minor flaws of the nose, never enhance the character of the face; their effect is always aging. The correction is indicated when you must worry about lighting so your bags won't show, when you feel more comfortable in dim light than daylight, and when your time with make-up is spent trying to hide your eyes' defects rather than highlight their assets. Blepharoplasty can turn an eyesore into an eyeful. It can turn someone's glance into a gaze.

Q&A

Will the operation interfere with my vision?

Temporarily, for the swelling and bruising from the surgery together with the eye-watering will cause some blurring. As these subside, visual acuity is restored to normal.

Am I blindfolded after surgery?

Most surgeons do not blindfold patients after surgery. It frightens many and prevents the surgeon from knowing whether or not the patient has light perception after the operation. The swelling can be constrained somewhat by chips of ice inserted into "Baggies" or plastic gloves that are placed over the lids.

Will a blepharoplasty change the shape of my eyes?

Unless you request a "sloe" or "doe" look, the conventional blepharoplasty will not change the shape of your eyes.

Can I wear glasses right after eyelid surgery?

The first day, no. By the second day, you may wear reading or dark glasses. If you wear contact lenses, they should not be worn until approximately five or six days after surgery.

Can I be put to "sleep" when I have this operation?

Yes, but it is not recommended. The exactness of this procedure leaves little margin for error. Under local analgesia there is still facial tone in force during the surgery and this helps guide the surgeon as to how much tissue to remove, whereas a slack face under a general anesthetic leaves too much to chance. A general anesthetic also subjects the patient to more risk and usually increased bleeding, which can interfere with any artistic endeavor.

4
The Face and Neck: Give Them A Raise

From time immemorial people have been identified by their faces. This emblem, unfortunately, displays the hallmarks of aging sooner and more vividly than any other organ. It is really not surprising that corruption of the facial skin often produces a greater lament than the more degenerative biochemical aspects of aging, especially among women. Aging may be man's destiny, but for women it is also their vulnerability.

This destiny can be a harrowing journey, one that affects all mankind in similar ways. Although the tempo of aging is different for each of us, the ever-changing scenery is much the same. Youth races past quickly enough, but old age comes at a gallop. It seems that we have not yet finished being young when we are already beginning to be old.

Meet Evelyn

She was a forty-year-old white female who came to my office requesting a face-lift. Happily married and strictly a family woman, she had woven the fabric of her life around her husband and three children. Throughout her married years she had taken care of them, and in so doing, had sadly neglected herself. Now the children were grown and leaving home. She had paused, taken a long look of self-appraisal, and was not happy with what the merciless years had done to her face.

Although her husband loved her as she was, he was appreciative of her concern and promised the operation for her forty-fifth birthday. He was ten years older than she, but appeared younger. She wanted to keep pace with him and viewed the operation more akin to self-preservation than pandering to human vanity.

Examination revealed a rather thin, attractive female. Facially, the engraving of time and gravity distinctly showed. Her youthful jaw line had been lost due to the skin slack, and there were numerous lines and furrows about the lips. Her severest problem was at the front of her neck, which was crepelike. Sagging downward, hammock-fashion, from her chin were several vertical folds that destroyed the clean chin-neck line.

Since she was in excellent health, the operation was scheduled as an office procedure, and it was a face saver! A small incision was placed beneath the chin enabling the surgeon to identify and eradicate the turkey-gobbler folds. The face-lift was performed to clean up the face and remainder of the neck. Four days later when the bandage was discarded, the swelling was minimal. The area around her mouth was then peeled and covered with adhesive tape. The next day the tape was removed and the area dusted with medicinal powder. By the eighth day her facial swelling and bruising were nonexistent, and the crust was flaking away from her lips. On the twelfth day, except for a red incision line under her chin and a very red area around her lips, it was difficult to tell she had had an operation.

When she returned for a postoperative visit after three months she looked radiant. She said: "Before it was like decorating an old Christmas tree. All the highlights in the world never made it look fresh and new. Now just a touch of make-up lights up my face."

Aging—What's In It For You?

Most of us dislike the idea of growing old. More honest would be the frank admission that this dislike is largely fear. As we grow old, the sense of death becomes a reality to all of us. Among all the creatures on the face of the earth, only man has a well-developed sense of time. He alone is cursed with the knowledge of finiteness and the awareness that someday he will cease to be. Thus, the reason we fear age is not that it kills us, but that once it makes its appearance, we know the length of the fuse.

Women, in particular, view aging as an impending doom, for they are also penalized as they pass their prime. This is not true for men, who rarely panic about getting older in the way many women do. Because our culture is more accepting of older men, there is a double standard: aging can enhance a man's image. He can attract a much younger woman. For women, the advancing years bring few rewards; our society counts physical attractiveness and youth much more important for women than men. If widowed or divorced in her later years, a woman may find it difficult to remarry someone her own age. Thus aging often means a gradual, degrading process of sexual disqualification since women are considered at their most eligible when youthful, after which their sexual value drops steadily. In essence, they are old as soon as they no longer look very young.

We live in a country where new is good and old is bad. Because old age is bad, the mature often feel inferior to the young. In its obsession with youth, our society labels people as socially old by removing them from their customary employment at the age of sixty-five, despite evidence that a person's level of mentality is maintained well past seventy; the country's Chief Executive has often been beyond the magic sixty-five. Upon retirement, their intellectual reservoir goes with them, wiping out years of experience. Because they lose the stimulus of feeling useful, this rejection based on age, or just an aged appearance, can be a deadly assault to their ego.

Looking for Immortality

The search for ways to prolong life or recapture lost youth has long been a staple of myth and folklore. Biblical kings indulged in the practice of sleeping with young virgins in order to absorb revitalizing emanations from their bodies—a treatment that, if it did nothing else, certainly made them happy and kept them from being lonely. Trojan warriors consumed the marrow of young bears to increase their strength and courage. And Asian physicians around 800 B.C. advised impotent patients to eat the testes of tigers. Even today, gerontologists and rejuvenation specialists conduct thriving practices, sometimes using techniques that are hardly less bizarre.

For all of medicine's skills, old age is as inevitable today as it was thousands of years ago. Scientists still cannot pinpoint when it begins because there is such variability in humans. A further complication is the fact that physiologic aging varies not only from person to person, but even within the same individual. Thus, eyesight can fail while the hearing mechanism remains perfect. In other words, a person can be at different ages within his own body in terms of physical and mental health.

Gerontology, the branch of science that deals with the aging process, has been sadly neglected in medical research, and is still in its infancy. We remain quite ignorant of the helter-skelter nature of aging and of the factors that accelerate or retard its erratic course. We know little of its biochemistry. In fact, aging is a process so little understood that it is a weak hook upon which to hang the cloak of disorders or diseases. Old age even resists precise definition; no common denominator for the condition has ever been found. Is it feeling old and tired or looking haggard and wrinkled? Is it chronological, physiological, psychological, or a combination of these?

Why we die is an even greater riddle since the human fabric is capable of repairing itself to a remarkable degree and mortality can only be explained with philosophic speculation. Possibly the mammalian cell contains a built-in clock so that there is a time for living and a time for dying. Some think of life itself as a deadly disease only cured by death; although cosmetic surgery has taken issue with time and has, for many, forced the clock to tick more slowly, medical science has not yet vanquished death, which lends a democratic cast to the face of all mankind.

The Range of Facial Change

Although medical specialists still have not determined what ignites the deterioration, the average person is all too aware of what the fire does to his body. Four major differences set the old face apart from the young one: changes in the color of the skin (see chapter 5); changes in the skull, which becomes thinner through bone absorption and occupies less volume (in other words, it shrinks); natural lines of expression of the face and neck deepen and become more apparent; and the skin sags into bags, jowls, pouches, and wattles because of the loss of elasticity and atrophy of fat, plus the effects of gravity.

These changes are most pronounced around the eyelids, the corners of the mouth and nose, and at the front of the neck. As this quiet, endless tragedy unfolds, the face seems ultimately to melt under the harrowing march of time.

To try and stop this melting process, we invest in creams and lotions, hormones and massages, and packs and other esoteric devices purchasable at apothecaries, health spas, beauty salons, and rejuvenating clinics. Creams and lotions can soften and lubricate dry and roughened skin; health spas may firm your figure and hormones can improve your disposition; the "success" of rejuvenation therapy is still based mainly on testimonials rather than scientific facts. In the long term, none of these has proven effective in eradicating the principal signs of aging—wrinkles, jowls, and loose, hanging skin. Only an operation known as rhytidoplasty, or face-lift, has been able to achieve a satisfactory illusion of youth.

A Shift in Time Can Give You A Lift

For thousands of people, their face is their fortune; for thousands more, it is their misfortune. And countless others find it disturbing when they see the loose, sagging skin and deep facial lines that proclaim their loss of youth. If the face can be called an open book, then the tale told by the ravaged face can be a gothic horror story. Since old age is our universal adversary, there is no facial correction that can bring us such profound happiness and exquisite mental relief as the removal of the outward signs of aging. Although youth does give a certain freshness to beauty, a face-lift recharges the emotions, injects new confidence, and challenges the belief that a blooming and attractive appearance is confined only to the very young.

A host of misconceptions regarding the face-lift procedure has accumulated since the surgery was first performed around the turn of the century. Most common is the concept that merely stretching the skin offers lasting, substantial results. Skin is elastic and if simply stretched backward into a new position, will soon revert to its old posture. A lift that depends solely on skin removal (a "mini" lift) is certain to sag more readily, with wide scarring at the incision line (Figure 4-1).

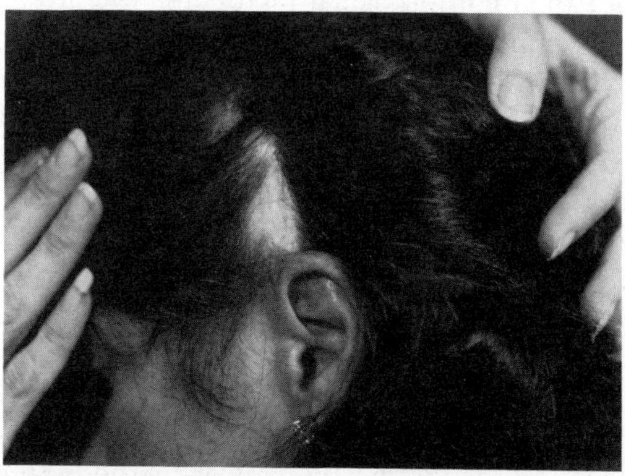

Figure 4-1 Wide scar producing a bald area—six months postoperative.

Mini lifts not only yield mini results, but are temporary, and leave the imprint of the surgeon's work for all to see. It is these procedures that have given rise to the stories of face-lifts suddenly falling overnight.

To visualize the marvels of a face-lift, many people place their fingers alongside the cheek area and pull the skin backwards. Their appearance is dramatically improved, but an incision (and resulting visible scar) would be intolerable in that area. The usual face-lift incision is located in the temple hairline well back from the facial region. When the fingers are placed in this area and exert a backward pull, it becomes evident that this approach will not accomplish significant changes. The "cleansing" effect gained in rhytidoplasty is achieved not by stretching, but by separating, *shifting* and *rotating* the skin and tissues of the face and neck. Thus, the proper procedure involves *shift* much more than lift.

With the increased understanding that a face-lift is the only effective technique to counter generalized sagging of the face and neck, much of the prejudice formerly surrounding this operation has been quelled. Not only is it used by movie stars, entertainers, and former First Ladies, but also by women (and men) in all walks of life. The remarkable youthful effects achieved have also brought this surgery out of the medical shadow-world. In the past decade, it has risen to become the third most popular cosmetic operation.

When should a face-lift be performed? At what age? Actually there is no age range for undergoing face-lift surgery. Determining when to perform a face-lift is primarily based on aesthetic rather than chronological factors. If you are chronologically young, but aesthetically old, and are disturbed by it, that is the time to contemplate surgery. It is much more rational to have surgery when the process of facial deterioration begins than to wait until the face is severely damaged by time. A face-lift performed at a younger age is better tolerated by the patient and is much more effective in its final result. It is actually easier to undergo surgery to keep from appearing older than to resort to it when old in an attempt to look younger.

The surgeon must rid the patient of her anxiety that if she undergoes surgery, she may need another face-lift in the future. Indeed, she very well may, as most of us will get older before we get any younger. The face, like the rest of the body, requires regular maintenance if it is to retain its youthfulness and vitality. The rationale of waiting for the sagging to become worse before having something done makes as much sense as having one dental cavity and waiting until there are ten before consulting a dentist. Why wait until it becomes worse? You may be dead by then! One should always live for the present, for that is the heart and soul of effective living.

The success of a face-lift largely depends on certain physical characteristics. The most satisfactory results can be expected from those who have high cheekbones and thin, sagging skin which is not oily, fat, or scarred, and retains a degree of elasticity. This thin, dry skin may quickly transmit bruising following surgery, but lends itself to classic improvement. Thick skin riddled with fat is like a big bedspread draped over a small cot. Unless the bedspread shrinks, it won't look attractive. Also, a full, fat face

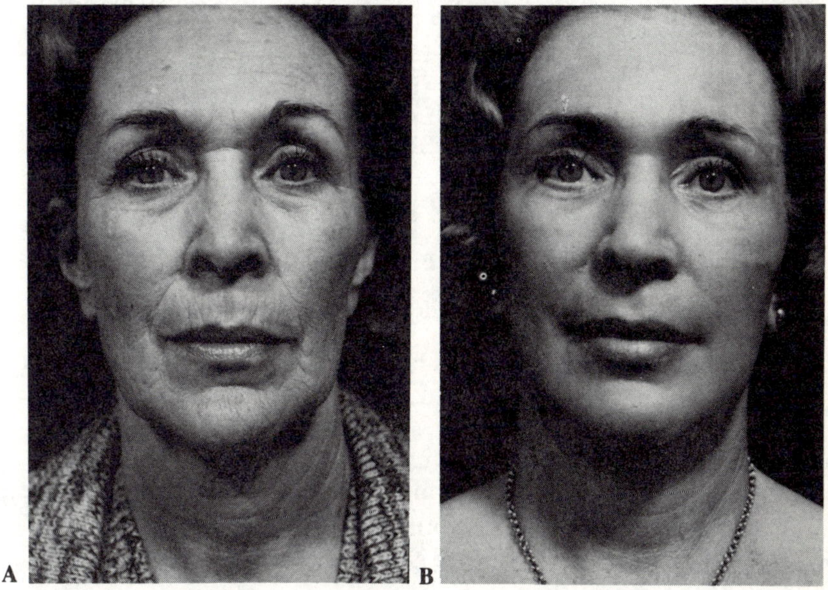

Figure 4-2 A. Facial skin demonstrating both sagging and diffuse wrinkling. **B.** Lift performed first followed by peel two months later. The combined procedures yield a smooth, tight appearance—one year postoperative.

does not permit easy shifting and rotation or a durable result, because the pull of gravity is greater; thus, the face-lift operation can fall short of its intended effect.

Approximately three quarters of the patients requesting a face-lift have deep lines and wrinkles that also require chemosurgery, known popularly as a face peel (see chapter 5). A face-lift is performed first to remove the gravitational sag and some of the wrinkles. If needed, a complete face peel is performed approximately six to eight weeks later, when most of the swelling has disappeared and the circulation has returned to normal (Figure 4-2). Spot peels (around the lips and forehead) can be

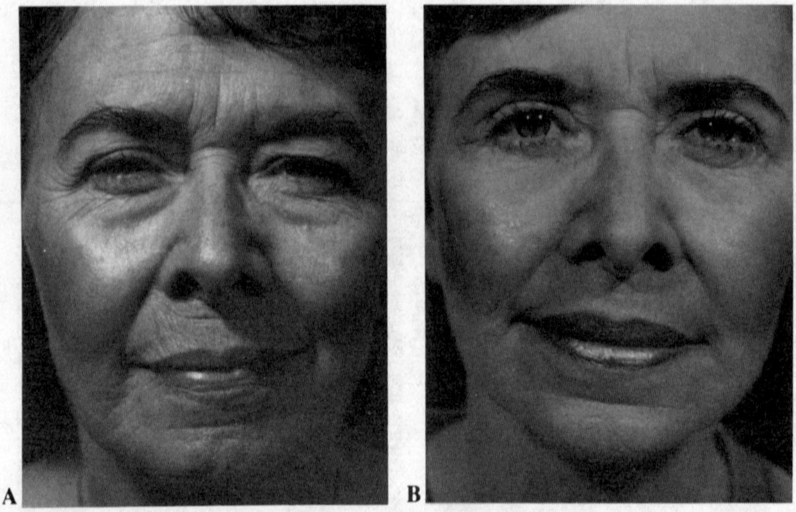

Figure 4-3 A. Facial sagging and eyelid drooping associated with abundant wrinkles. However, only wrinkles around the mouth disturbed the patient. **B.** Circumoral peel performed ten days after the lift—two months postoperative.

performed one week after surgery (Figure 4-3).

In certain patients, a drooping nasal tip can be corrected during the lift surgery to give a more youthful look. As stated in chapter 3, however, eyelid and face-lift procedures yield superior results when done separately.

How Is It Done?

Preoperative preparation for the lift is not elaborate. The patient's hair is shampooed the evening preceding the operation. Cleansing permits a minimum amount of hair to be trimmed at the incision sites and provides insurance against wound contamination by hair. The day of the surgery, the patient is sedated, taken to the operating room, prepped, and draped.

The face-lift operation involves incisions in the temporal

hairline which trace along the crease just in front of the ear (preauricular crease),* curve beneath the earlobe into the postauricular groove, and slope into the hairline at the back of the neck. All incisions and subsequent scars are either hidden by the hair or camouflaged in the natural creases in front and back of the ear (Figure 4-4).

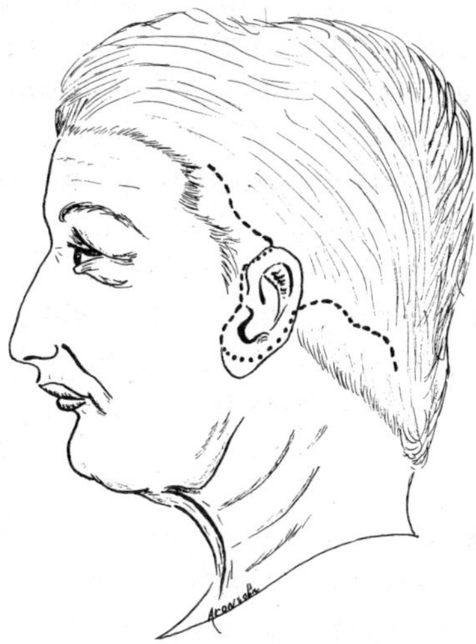

Figure 4-4 The incisions are hidden in the hair and in the deep recess behind the ear. The incision in front of the ear is camouflaged by the crease that is normally there in most people—the incision is the same for men and women.

After making the incision, the surgeon separates the skin from the underlying musculature and creates a large facial-neck flap. It is the release of the skin from the underlying tissues and its higher repositioning that endow the face-lift technique with its effectiveness. The underlying musculature in the face and neck is also shifted upward to create a new, firm bed for the overlying skin. Without this preparation, the skin shifting process would be comparable to the smoothing of a bedspread over rumpled blankets. The surgeon then rotates this large flap, shifts it upward

**Although some surgeons advocate placing the incision within the cartilaginous protrusion in front of the ear (the tragus), the preauricular incision should never be placed there. If a high tragus is present, as it is in most patients, normal wound contraction will distort this anatomical feature. This will not occur immediately, but within several months the tragus will be pulled down and flattened to give an unnatural look.*

and backward, and removes the excess skin.

The two halves of the face are not repaired simultaneously but in sequence—first, one side, then the other. As if creating a new design, the physician drapes and tailors the skin on each side to fit the face.

Upon occasion, if excessive fat is present along the jaw line, it is trimmed to give a more lean appearance. As this fat overlies important motor nerves that are responsible for facial tone, the surgeon must exercise great care during this maneuver; injury to these nerves will, literally, cause the patient to lose face. The facial paralysis that can ensue causes an emotionally devastating functional loss. An individual's face, together with its expressions, is his center of communication with the surrounding world.

Approximately one-and-a-half to two hours are necessary for a face-lift operation, depending upon the skill and experience of the surgeon and the pathology present. A "twilight sleep" analgesic is usually administered, thus eliminating the need for a general anesthetic which can be dangerous to some patients. It also constrains bleeding because of the adrenalin component that is mixed with the local.

This surgery, at one time confined only to the hospital, is now standard as an office procedure. Ambulatory surgical facilities offer significant cost savings to the patient (most insurance policies do not cover the operation) while assuring optimal use of hospital beds.

Forehead wrinkles can be satisfactorily corrected by surgical intervention, but their removal may be short-lived. Freeing the forehead skin from its underlying muscle, although it can achieve a smooth surface, offers no long-term smoothness unless a large portion of the frontal (forehead) muscle is removed. Both the sliding action of the scalp over the skull and the formation of wrinkles from contraction of the frontal muscles prohibit lasting improvement through any stretching process. Also, when the forehead is drawn upward and the excess skin is cut away, the frontal hairline is elevated, disturbing the normal relationship of the forehead with the rest of the face. This procedure should be limited to those individuals with a low frontal hairline. In selected cases, chemosurgery (described in chapter 5) offers a satisfactory result.

Frown furrows and lines also resist any lasting correction. They can be ameliorated, however, by droplets of silicone fluid, that initiate the formation of collagen and scar tissue between the skin and muscle. This scar formation, in selected cases, can soften these lines. Much depends upon the configuration and contour of the furrows as well as the type of skin, that is whether it is dry or oily, thick or thin, smooth or porous. This method demands great care; otherwise we pay too high a price in the poor coin of discoloration, prominent bulging, and permanent swelling around the tissues.

Furrows can also be softened by interrupting or removing the muscles that control the frown reflex. This is performed through a surgical approach across the hairline of the scalp at the same time that frontal wrinkles are being removed. However, with continuous, frequent frowning, any remaining muscle can hypertrophy, and the lines and furrows will return. Only by destroying the nerve to this muscle can frowns be surrendered forever. As this procedure denervates the muscles and sacrifices the patient's ability to express emotion by forehead gestures, it robs the face of natural expression. In time, this loss of muscle function can also cause the brows to droop. It is not, therefore, prescribed.

Some patients, besides having jowls and folds that hang from the jawline, also have large, fatty deposits under the chin. Despite dieting and exercise, the fat can linger tenaciously, spoiling the otherwise clean, pleasing chin-neck line. In most cases, the conventional face-lift alleviates the neck wattle and fat pad under the chin. However, if a vast amount of fat and sag is present, mere backward, lateral, and upward rotation of the skin without removal of fat accomplishes little change. Removal of the adipose tissue via the created facial flaps entails some danger to the motor nerves of the face as the dissection distance from the usual face-lift incisions is great and the visibility is also poor. A safer technique, and one that yields greater improvement, consists of attacking the problem through a normal crease found just beneath the chin. Through this incision, the fat is easily removed along with the redundant skin. From this site, the surgeon can also remove any unneeded neck cords (muscles) that may be present or sew them together, depending on the severity of the situation. The ready access and resulting youthful appearance warrants this separate incision and resulting fine scar, which is hidden from direct view by the chin.

In general, the neck alone should not be lifted; both the neck and face should be treated together. Otherwise there will be a tight neck under a generally sagging face, and it will not look natural. However, as an isolated procedure in young people who require just removal of fat or have slight sag in the neck when the rest of the face is firm, this procedure is ideal in obtaining a clean, definitive neckline.

After the Raise

Following the face-lift, the patient's head is wrapped in circumferential (encircling) bandages to maintain pressure on the newly shifted skin flaps. These bandages hinder the swelling and inhibit bleeding that might otherwise occur beneath the skin. This bulky dressing is removed on the following morning, and a smaller, more comfortable one applied. The second bandage is not disturbed until the fourth postoperative day, when it is taken off and the stitches in front of the ears are removed. Thereafter, no further bandaging is necessary. Healing proceeds rapidly in the preauricular areas, which are virtually devoid of tension. In the neck and temple areas, where the greatest tension exists, the healing process is slower, and the sutures are left in longer, about ten days.

Since each individual reacts differently to surgery, some will have more swelling and bruising than others. But it never happens as it does in movies, with the aging actress unraveling the bandages and looking radiant. Living tissue is being cut, bruised, stretched, and shaped. There is no way that this can be accomplished without some discomfort, swelling, and discoloration. As a rule, however, the swelling subsides substantially within five to seven days and by two weeks, most patients are fairly presentable and can return to work. In one month, the majority of patients are comfortably back within the mainstream of society without any sign of surgery.

If the operation is performed in a hospital, the patient can be treated as an outpatient or can remain in the hospital two to three days, depending on the patient, the surgeon, and the region of the country where the surgery took place. If the face-lift is an office procedure, the patient remains in recovery until fully conscious; then she can be taken home. Minimal care is needed that evening. There are no diet restrictions with a face-lift, and primary concern is directed toward administering medication to relieve pain and permit sleep.

For the first two weeks, the doctor sees the patient weekly. During this immediate convalescent period, you must curtail some activities to ensure adequate healing. Although a bath the first postoperative day is permissible, do not shower until the fourth postoperative day, when the bandage is discarded. You may shampoo your hair at this time. Some sutures will still be present, but gentle shampooing will not harm or infect them. Do not have your hair tinted until three weeks after surgery. A wig may be worn within two weeks. While bandaged, wash the exposed part of your face with a sudsy facecloth, being careful not to wet the bandage. Once the bandage is off, you can cleanse the entire face, using caution around the incision lines so as not to disrupt them. Male patients may shave by the fifth day. By the fourth postoperative day, most patients can drive, and after three weeks they may resume other outside activities, although they should avoid exposing the face to direct sunlight for approximately one month.

Patients may experience occasional shooting pains and numbness over the neck, face, and about the ear lobes. All this is a part of the normal process of healing and should disappear in approximately six weeks. Do not wear earrings until sensation in the lobes returns. The lines of incision remain red for several months, but as healing progresses they blanch out. Makeup and hair styling can conceal these during the healing phase.

Complications are rare in a rhytidoplasty; the face is imbued with a rich vascularity that thwarts infection. Bruising does occur beneath the skin following the surgery, but is not a serious problem. The large head bandage inhibits any massive collection of blood beneath the flap, an accumulation that could endanger the viability of the skin and produce ulcerations.

The temple and nape scars (located within the hair) should be minimal if more shift than lift is employed. This maneuver will also minimize the possibility of hair loss in these areas. However, should hair loss occur, hair transplants can rectify the situation. Cortisone injections can flatten thickened scars. The preauricular scar is usually very fine as the skin is reattached here with virtually no tension. Black people should be forewarned that despite all precautions, hypertrophic scarring can occur along any of the incisions.

Notwithstanding all articles to the contrary, it is impossible to end up with a tight, mask-like appearance if the face is lifted and drawn too tightly because facial movements are controlled by muscles and not by skin. The skin, which is intimately attached to the underlying muscles, is merely a drape and moves in unison with muscle contraction. If the muscles or their nerves have not been damaged, facial expression will not be disturbed. For a few days, while there is some swelling and bruising, the face may have a tense or rigid appearance, but as the swelling subsides, the expression will return to normal. What can happen, however, if the skin is reattached too tightly, is that the incision site will act like any scar under tension—it will spread and, instead of a fine line, the patient will be left with a broad, thick scar. Excessive tension in the temple and neck can also endanger the blood supply of the skin in these areas, leading to ulcerations and loss of hair.

A widespread myth endows the face-lift with the power to create beauty. A face-lift's sole purpose is to make one appear younger; as it leaves the bony architecture untouched and does nothing to improve the facial texture, only a measure of the beauty that once existed can be regained. In fact, the process of erasing age should be subtle, not blatant. The surgeon should remove the old rather than strive to make the person look young. Otherwise, the patient can emerge with a certain "plastic" appearance.

Will It Last?

Contrary to a popular opinion stating that once you have had a face-lift, you must keep having them, the opposite is true. For when the skin is freed and moved into a new position, the scar that forms between it and the underlying tissues binds it in place and prevents it from sliding as easily as before. Also, the result will not collapse overnight. In other words, if you are fifty-five years old and the operation makes you look forty-five, ten years from now, with proper care, you will look fifty-five, not sixty-five.

It is difficult to predict how long the facial improvement will last, nor should the surgeon ever tell patients that they will look a certain number of years younger. The surgeon who does so may be hanging from a slender branch. Such predictions lie within the realm of clairvoyance, not science. Since appraisal of results is highly subjective, if not emotional, what surgeon can possibly be mathematically precise about how much younger a patient will appear? Duration depends upon so many variables such as genetic factors, skin elasticity, physical health, and stability of weight, among others. What the surgeon does is take the patient back a certain number of years to a new baseline. How well the patient ages then depends primarily on the person's mode of living and how well she takes care of herself.

For both physiological and psychological reasons, a face-lift can be disappointing. The operation is not a permanent correction. And quite often, we are dealing with more than just the aging process. It may be a time of great frustrations, worries, and disillusionments and many patients expect the surgery to alleviate these emotional problems.

Some patients complain that after several months their face begins to sag again and why wasn't more skin taken away? At the time of surgery, all the slack that is safe to remove is removed. As was stated, to draw up the skin too tightly can lead to broad scarring, loss of hair, and ulcerations at the wound edges. Postoperative weight fluctuations, twisting, rotating, and the taffy-pull that skin is subjected to all take their toll. Many patients have sought the operation after undertaking crash diets that have depleted their body's protein, leading to wasting, thinning, and atrophic changes in the muscles, skin, and fat. It is unreasonable to expect tissues not adequately nourished to respond favorably to undermining, shifting, stretching, or manipulation.

There are cases where a sustained reducing diet will make for better face-lift results. The nasolabial line (the line or fold running down from the corner of the nose) is a smile line, and is a case in point. It is very difficult to correct or remove; at best, it

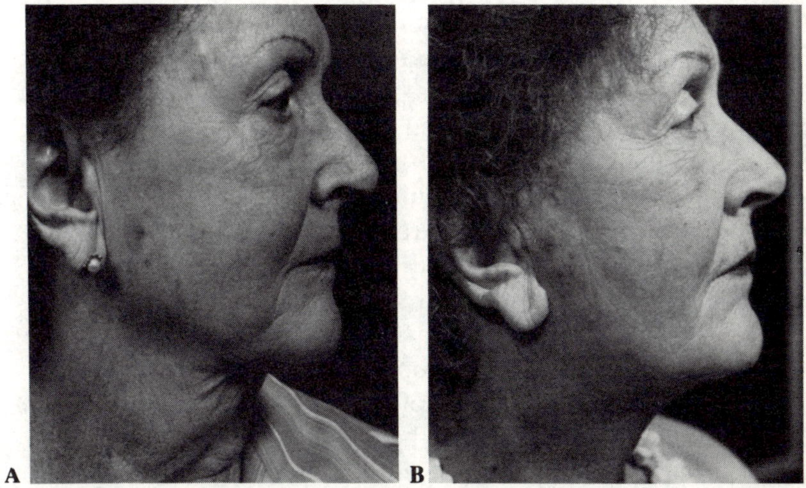

Figure 4-5 A. Generalized sagging of face with marked wrinkling and excess skin of the neck. **B.** Ten days postoperative; note how even and smooth the neck appears.

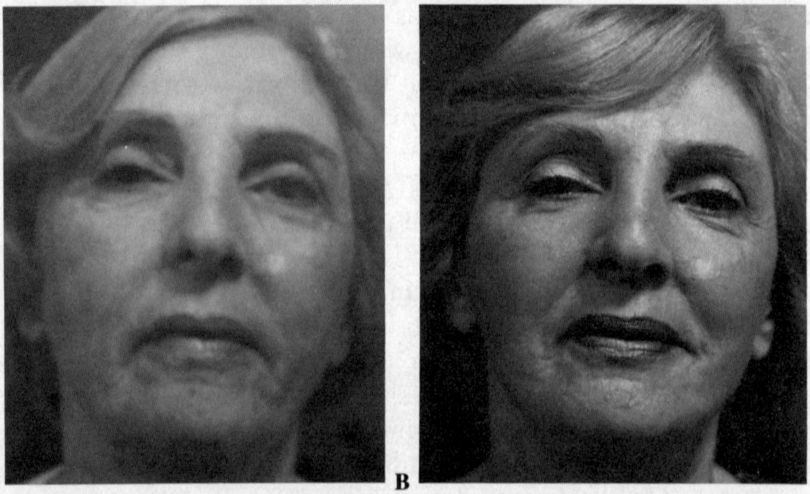

A B

Figure 4-6 **A.** Numerous lines, wrinkles and facial sagging. **B.** A face-lift followed by facial chemosurgery (peeling) several months later—five months postpeel, seven months postoperative.

can be softened. This fold is more prevalent in obese patients and in these individuals particularly, the face-lift operation will not yield consummate improvement. They should participate in a sensible reducing program prior to surgery.

Whatever the duration, the person who has been made to look younger by a face-lift will continue to look younger as the years go by and will never look as old as he or she would have without the operation. Figures 4-5, 4-6, and 4-7 demonstrate the improvement achieved with this surgery.

How often can you have a face-lift? Certainly the surgery does not stop one from aging. Aging is relentless. A lift merely shifts the "aesthetic clock" backward and the patient begins aging from a new point in time. Thus, if facial sagging and redundant skin recur, one can have as many lifts as necessary unless health barriers intervene. Each time the operation is performed, the old scars are removed so that one is not left with any additional scars. With each lift, the amount of hair-bearing skin removed is relatively scant, and little change will be noted in the hairline. Even when the hairline is moderately set back, it will not draw attention if symmetry is maintained between the two halves of the face.

As for cost, the average fee for a rhytidoplasty is about $3500;

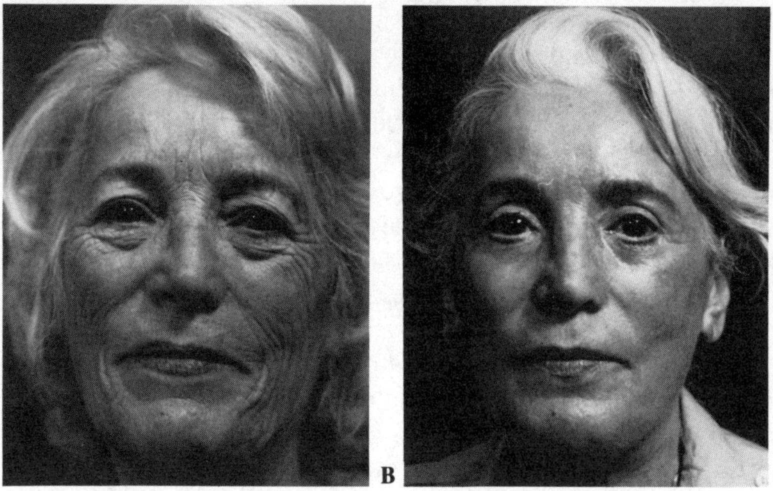

A B

Figure 4-7 A. Severe wrinkling of face together with sagging eyelid and facial areas. **B.** Final result after eyelid and facial surgery followed by facial chemosurgery one year later—two years postsurgery and one year post peel.

however, a wide range exists—from $2500 to $5000, depending on the surgeon's experience and reputation. The cost of silicone injections averages $50 per treatment, more or less at the discretion of the physician. Insurance plans rarely help to pay for a face-lift. The cost, however, may be deducted (as all cosmetic surgeries can) as a medical expense on income tax returns.

The March of Time

As mentioned earlier, the acid of time is more corrosive for women than for men; the face-lift operation has mainly been associated with them. While lines and wrinkles in men confer an image of virility, in women they bestow no sexual illusion. They merely foreshadow the onset of old age. A man's face is something he basically doesn't need to tamper with; all he has to do is keep it clean. He can also, if he wants, hide behind his beard. By contrast, a woman's face is potentially separate from her body and she does not treat it naturalistically. As Oscar Wilde once stated: "A man's face is his autobiography; a woman's face is her work of fiction."

Yet this situation is changing, as evidenced by the increasing number of men who have face-lifts. The surgery does pose a slight problem for men because of their sideburns and beards. With the shifting of the skin, hair-bearing segments along the jaw and neck may end up behind the ear. This can be corrected during surgery by destroying the hair follicles along the shifted beard line; alternatively, the follicles can be removed later by electrolysis.

During the past fifty years, there has been a change in the age distribution of our population. The fall in the birth rate and the decline in the death rate have caused a proportional shift in the ratio of young people to old. Today more than 40 percent of Americans are over forty-five. Twenty million are now over sixty-five. Conservative estimates indicate that, by 1990, 27 million people in the United States will be over 65. America is turning gray, but we are not ready for it.

This increase in the number of older people is producing bewildering sociological, economic, and psychological problems. For many of us no longer grow old gracefully. We dwell mainly on old age's somber side. Nor does our society always value experience. Instead of using the wisdom of age to help solve our problems, we have turned the aged themselves into a problem. Our fascination with youth has made us forget that often, people considered "too old" have the youngest ideas of all.

Although there is no period of life without its particular pain, being old and looking it is exceptional in its torment and is regarded as the Achilles' heel of the American system. In today's highly competitive world, with its ubiquitous youth cult, there is a seeming conspiracy against the aged. The word itself has been purged. We speak not of old people but of "senior citizens." The elderly are often hidden from the rest of society in bleak, overcrowded sanitariums, or in geriatric ghettos, to become in many cases, rocking-chair prisoners. Medical advances are keeping them alive at the same time that technology is making them obsolete. Old age is the ultimate test of an individual's courage, dignity, and talent. In many cases, it brings sadness not because it signals the end of enjoyment, but because it marks the end of hope. Here death is not a tragedy, but merely an anticlimax.

When we are young, so many of us are too busy to appreciate fully the meaning of life. We wish to advance and achieve success. Because of this drive for success, we exchange youth for attainment. By the time we've attained what we've struggled for, the years of strife and travail have left their indelible mark.

Because we are terribly preoccupied in this country not just with age, but with how old a person looks, many people consider it a biological injustice that the outward signs of deterioration become evident virtually at the height of their mental, physical, and economic maturity. Few people feel their age; they only look it. Since many young minds are masked behind old faces, partial relief is available through a face-lift.

When charm, experience, and glamor cannot counterbalance the total visual effects of capricious genes, time, weather, and stress, another formidable weapon is equal to the challenge. Today's female need not suffer the erosion of her femininity, nor spend her life spinning fantasies till *The Iceman Cometh*. She no longer has to wind up as unwanted or as wilted as yesterday's salad; the cosmetic surgeon, a real knight of today, can rescue her. Although the scalpel has replaced the lance, the deliverance can be just as dramatic.

Q&A

Will I need to keep having a face-lift once I have one?

That depends on your point of view. Aging will continue and to maintain that illusion of youth you may need further redraping, resurfacing (peeling), and replacement (silicone, collagen) therapy.

Will my face look unnatural and mask-like after my lift?

A face-lift makes the face taut by cutting away the skin excess and by firming up the superficial muscles beneath the skin. If the muscles and their nerves are not damaged, your facial expression will be natural since the skin is intimately attached to the muscles and is merely a drape over them. Stretching the skin too tightly may give a masklike look for a short time, but the real danger is elsewhere. The elastic skin will soon revert to its previous site, leaving wide scars and baldness in its wake.

Will my face suddenly fall back to what it was overnight?

No—any lift that is based on shifting rather than stretching should be lasting. This implies that the skin is freed from its underlying muscles and redraped upward. As the skin heals, it fastens itself into this new position and aging begins from this new posture.

When is the best age to have a face-lift?

There is none exactly. Determination of when to have a lift is based on aesthetic rather than on chronological age. If you are thirty years old but look haggard and much older, then now is the best time for a lift. The greatest number of lifts, however, are performed when the patients are in their forties and fifties, as that is the usual time that gravity first begins to display its forces markedly.

How long will a lift last?

That is so variable from patient to patient, it is impossible to give a clear answer. Aging is also variable from one person to another and what will last in one may not be so lasting in another. Remember, a lift removes the excess skin and shifts upward what remains so the face looks more taut. The operation does nothing to restore the skin's elasticity which may be more vital in one patient than another. This vitality alone lends itself to a more lasting correction. Only diamonds are forever.

5
The Skin—You're Right Behind It

The skin plays a most significant role in our lives. It not only reflects the shape of the body and transmits its sensations, but it is also our principal medium of sexual attraction. We can cold-cream it, suntan it, bleach it, lift it, and paint it—but we literally cannot shed it. Skin is the mirror that reflects our health, whether good or bad. Skin is alive; it grows and repairs itself continuously. Skin is versatile; it secretes sweat and oil, regulates body temperature and blood flow, and reacts to temperature and touch. Skin is variable: it can be white or black, soft or rough, thick or thin, smooth or hairy. Our most obvious personal characteristic, our physical appearance, is predominantly due to our skin.

What's in the Skin for You?

Wrapping us as it does from head to foot, skin constitutes the largest organ of the body. And behind this thin anatomical sheath simmers a veritable hive of activity. The skin is the agent for reception of touch, pain, and temperature and is richly furnished with sensory nerves for the performance of these duties. By virtue of conduction, radiation, and evaporation from its surface, the skin ranks as an important element in the process of temperature regulation (dilation of the capillary networks allows a greater blood flow through the skin, thus cooling the body; a lesser flow warms the body). The underlying cushion of fat intimately connected with the skin not only acts as the guardian of body heat, but also functions as a shock absorber in case of injury. Although the skin performs these functions effortlessly and without parade, most of us regard and embellish it as merely a showcase.

The outer layer of skin, the epidermis, is an avascular, flaky layer of dead cells that can vary from thick (4 to 5 millimeters) over the palms and soles, to thin (0.5 millimeter) over the eyelids. It is nourished from below by the dermis, which is the true skin.. The dermis is a dense mass of elastic, interlacing tissue, riddled with fine blood vessels, nerves, roots of hairs, and glands for making sweat and oil. Sweat glands are particularly abundant on the palms, soles, and in the armpits and their secretion is dictated not only by temperature, but also by nervousness and anxiety. Oil glands are most abundant about the face and hair; they secrete an oily substance that prevents dryness and helps maintain a supple skin. These oil glands, although small and inert in childhood, become physiologically active at puberty and constitute one of the principal factors in acne vulgaris, discussed later in this chapter.

Skin color is determined at birth and cannot be altered under normal conditions. The human skin has a palette of five pigments sprawled between the two layers and applies them in various proportions to achieve assorted blends. Oxyhemoglobin (hemoglobin containing oxygen), found in the blood vessels, imparts a rosy glow; reduced hemoglobin (lacking oxygen), also in the blood vessels, give a bluish tint; carotene adds a creamy, golden tinge, especially to fatty terrain; and melanoid adds shadowy tones. Seen through the transparent surface cells, these pigments make the skin look pasty or pinkish white. Melanin, the fifth but most important tone on the palette, enhances this pasty blend to create the subtle light and dark variations of skin color.

It is difficult to judge whether black is beautiful or whether white is, for that matter. But one can unequivocally state that black is young. Darker-skinned people are less susceptible to the onslaught of the sun's rays in direct proportion to the amount of melanin in their skin. Black skin with its high melanin content affords natural protection against the sun because the pigment acts as a filter, absorbing and degrading the ultraviolet and actinic radiation so that far less of it gets through to the dermis and its vascular system. Thus, elderly blacks often appear deceptively young-looking.

The nature of the body's biochemistry that leads to aging of the skin is not completely understood, but like the tides, it is predictable and unrelenting. Between birth and death, the caucasian skin is transformed from a pink velvety finish to a yellow leathery surface—first wrinkles, then sagging that evolves into folds that gravitate downward into jowls, pouches, and wattles.

Lines and wrinkles are caused by the skin's loss of elasticity as the collagen and elastin fibers in the dermis become brittle and dried out. Also, the epidermis and dermis atrophy and become thin, causing the skin to forfeit its velvety texture and assume a lustreless tinge of yellow. The skin is further marred by pigmentation spots and many dilated blood vessels that easily peek through the thin outer layers.

Sagging is due to the decreased volume of the skull and its overlying fat and soft tissue, together with the loss of skin elasticity; thus, the skin becomes too large for the skull and tends to sag because of the slack.

Tanning May Look Beautiful, But . . .

Perhaps the most potent catalyst in the skin-aging process is overexposure to the sun's rays. Sufficient intensity of ultraviolet radiation penetrates the earth's atmosphere to damage all but the very dark-skinned. Although a tan imparts a feeling and an image of healthiness, the sun's rays inflict a deferred sorrow. This is particularly true for blue-eyed, fair-skinned persons. Ordinarily, it is the fair-haired, fair-skinned and light-eyed individual who develops deep wrinkles since he does not possess enough melanin to protect his skin from the sun's rays. Protection for the face is essential for these individuals as facial coloring is mainly due to the blood beneath the skin surface.

What protection can accomplish is vividly illustrated by examining the front part of the neck directly under the chin. The

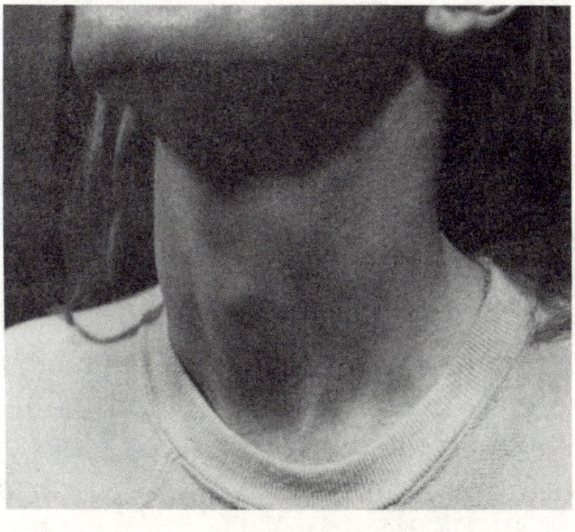

Figure 5-1 The unprotected skin appears veiny and pigmented compared to the smooth, white protected skin beneath the "V" of the chin.

shadow cast by the chin protects this V-shaped area from the sun's rays and the skin here is always smoother, whiter and lighter than the wrinkled, pigmented, and veiny skin surrounding it (Figure 5-1). Aged skin is diseased skin, which is in a large measure preventable.

The young in particular are notoriously incapable of foreseeing the consequences of careless or irrational behavior, especially if the penalty is delayed to some misty time in the future. It is unfortunate that the skin changes are not visible until decades after they have seriously begun. What may appear as mahogany at twenty will look like leather at forty, for over a period of years continued overexposure to sunlight can result in chemical breakdown and cellular damage of dermal tissue. That fine tan* will come back to haunt you and surface in the form of deep wrinkles, leathery folds, and pigmentations. As sunlight cruises through the atmosphere, it does not simply caress the skin, but marks it with a deadly touch.

Acne: Scars Are the Pits

The most common and most cosmetically distressing problem that the dermatologist sees in his office is the skin disease known as acne vulgaris. This disorder begins primarily during the adolescent's loss of innocence and awakening of sexual maturity, when concern with appearance and popularity is at its peak. Also, acne is often equated with being "dirty." It is little wonder that abnormal personality patterns, emotional anguish, and mental disturbances frequently occur in youngsters with this affliction.

Acne is primarily a problem of hormonal imbalance, which is genetically predetermined—you inherit the tendency to get it. Male hormones present in both sexes stimulate activity of the oil glands. Acne vulgaris strikes about ninety percent of men and seventy percent of women at some time in their lives and usually leaves distinctive tracks in its trail.

An imbalance in the female/male hormone ratio leads to a surplus of male hormone, which stimulates the oil glands within the hair follicle to excessive production. When too much oil is secreted too fast, it clogs the pores. These oil plugs darken (oxidize) on exposure to air, producing the characteristic

* *The production of pigment cells (melanin) is increased as a physiological response to ultraviolet light. After a prolonged stimulus, they form a thick, dark, protective layer over the more vulnerable cells; the darkened skin is called a tan.*

comedone (blackhead). Blocked comedones are the "time bombs" of acne for they obstuct the follicle drainage. The oil glands continue to secrete at a high rate, but the oil trapped beneath the surface stagnates and becomes inflamed, producing a pimple. As the inflammation continues, the pimple expands and bursts, forming a boil. The expanding infection destroys a region of healthy tissue, leaving a craterlike cavity that heals with scar-tissue formation. When the scar contracts (as all scars do), the skin surface is depressed, leaving characteristic pits in the scar's wake. The blemish can also be thick and raised in those individuals with a propensity for developing enlarged scars.

Will the Real Treatment for Acne Please Stand Up?

How do you treat acne? There are probably as many ways of treatment for this enigmatic skin disease as there are dermatologists dealing with it. All physicians agree that the patient should be educated to realize that treatment will be varied and will be long term. At this writing, there is no known definite cure for acne.

Because it is a hormonal problem, contraceptive pills are often administered. Sometimes the condition improves with these, but often it does not, and occasionally it even gets worse. Because of the pill's side effects physicians are prescribing it less frequently these days. For one of the side effects is another skin problem—blotching or hyperpigmentation (chloasma, mask of pregnancy) that worsens in sunlight. When induced by contraceptive pills, this reaction is more extensive than in normal pregnancy since the pills can be taken for more than nine months and this type of chloasma is very resistant to treatment.

Antibiotics can do wonders for acne, but may cause intestinal upsets by disturbing the bacterial equilibrium in the intestines. Many individuals develop severe allergies to antibiotics, with a reaction that may be worse than any possible benefit.

For years, various diets have been advocated for acne sufferers. Most physicians today agree that diet has little to do with causing the eruptions, although in certain instances some foods may cause flare-ups, most likely because of allergy or idiosyncrasy.

Repeated vigorous scrubbing of the face with soaps, abrasives, solvents, and lotions cleanses the face temporarily, but does not affect the inordinate activity of the oil glands. The application of liquid Vitamin A acid as well as many sulfur prescriptions does improve the skin by accelerating its normal peeling, thus removing the blemishes as the top layer is shed. However, these substances cause marked reddening and dryness of the skin, which are apparent and difficult to cover with make-up.

Although there is a myriad of ways to treat acne, there is no surefire method of treating the scars it causes. The newest method, one still under investigation, is by injecting purified liquid collagen underneath the pit, thus elevating it. Collagen is a fundamental protein of the body. Animal (bovine) collagen is liquefied and stripped of the antigens that cause tissue rejection when injected into a human. The human body thus accepts the material as belonging to itself, and the collagen becomes indistinguishable from the surrounding tissues and skin. To date this technique has shown great promise, especially in shallow, saucerlike scars caused by chickenpox and some cases of acne. Ice-pick type scars are not ameliorated by this method. Since collagen is a live, foreign protein, it may cause severe allergic reactions in those sensitive to bovine serum.

For twenty years, doctors have used liquefied silicone to elevate acne scars in the manner mentioned above. When injected, silicone stimulates the production of collagen. It will not move or migrate when used in proper amounts. Unlike bovine collagen, silicone is not a live protein and therefore is safer to inject. Despite this, some cases of marked foreign-body reaction have occurred, causing redness and lumps in the skin. Silicone treatment, like that of collagen, is also limited by the types of scars that are presented.

Fibrin foam, a component of blood, can also be used to elevate depressed scars. A small amount of the patient's blood is taken and, through a simple laboratory procedure, fibrin is extracted. The doctor then frees the scar surgically from its tissue below and injects the foam beneath to plump it up. Surgical glue closes the fine nick in the skin. No side effects, such as rejection or allergy, occur since the fibrin comes from the patient's body. Like collagen and silicone injections, it is an office procedure.

A time interval must elapse before repeating the procedure. Hence, there is a further degree of discomfort because blood must be redrawn each time, since fibrin foam becomes unstable after one week. Also, because the scar must be surgically elevated before the solution can be injected, it must be anesthetized. The procedure is tedious and prolonged. However, as scars are treated individually, the entire surface of the face is not involved; the process is therefore less expensive than dermabrasion.

A face-lift has been advocated by some surgeons as a method to ameliorate the diffuse shallow-type acne scars. They believe that freeing the scarred skin from the underlying tissue, then shifting it upward, will smooth and soften the scars. In theory it is reasonable. In practice it is not. In the majority of patients, the scars are merely shifted upward into a new position with minimal to no change in their form. This procedure is not recommended to help improve this type of scarring.

Dermabrasion

This Close "Shave" Will Help

Dermabrasion, also known as planing or sanding, is another timetested way of treating the scars caused by acne. It is a procedure that is far from ideal. For although abrasion can improve the face cosmetically, it will not leave a completely smooth skin. Acne pits develop from scarring at various depths below the epidermis and depress the skin. The goal in treating irregular surfaces is to sand down the high points or elevations so that the low ones appear less deep. Improvement occurs because once the dermis has been thinned by this technique, it never regains its original thickness. As the wound heals after an abrasion, a new layer of epidermis forms over the raw dermal surface. However, if one attempts to delve too deep in an effort to remove all the pits, the process itself can produce scarring.

Pores are not improved by dermabrasion or by any chemical or physical process that is known today. The true pore, quite different from the popular conception of a pore, is an opening of the sweat gland hidden within the skin. Our concern is with an external opening of the skin that is often called a pore, but is actually the inelastic surface opening of a hair follicle where no hair exists. The size of these pores is genetically predetermined. The puffing that follows either abrasion or peeling lessens their prominence for a while because of the swelling of the interpore skin structure. As the swelling subsides, the pores return as vivid as ever. They may in fact become worse since the hair follicle widens as it penetrates deeper into the skin; a deep abrasion, like a deep peel, can only make them more conspicuous.

Severe scarring from acne usually requires more than one planing and, although it can minimize the pits, planing rarely removes all their traces. When a second planing is indicated, it can, in most cases, be undertaken approximately six months after the first operation. Since it removes the entire epidermis where the pigment (melanin) resides, the abraded areas will have a lighter look which may not be noticeable in the fair-skinned (as their coloring is due mainly to their blood); it will be apparent in the dark-skinned and they should be so forewarned. The line of demarcation between the abraded and nonabraded skin resembles a continuous dirt line and is just below the jaw between the face and neck. It is partially hidden by the shadow of the jaw and makeup will further help the camouflage.

The face responds best to dermabrasion or peeling as it contains the highest density of regenerating tissue (hair follicles and sweat glands) and is imbued with a rich vascularity. The neck fares less well because it is thinner, less vascular, and contains less regenerating tissue. The chest and back react poorly from any attack and if abraded may heal slowly, poorly, and with manifest scars or keloid formation.

If only a small area of the face requires treatment, planing is generally performed in the surgeon's office under a local analgesic. Spot planing, however, produces a contrast in color between the planed and unplaned skin. It is better practice to sand the entire face for it then exhibits a pink glow overall.

It makes no difference if there are active lesions and eruptions present since planing performs a function similar to that of

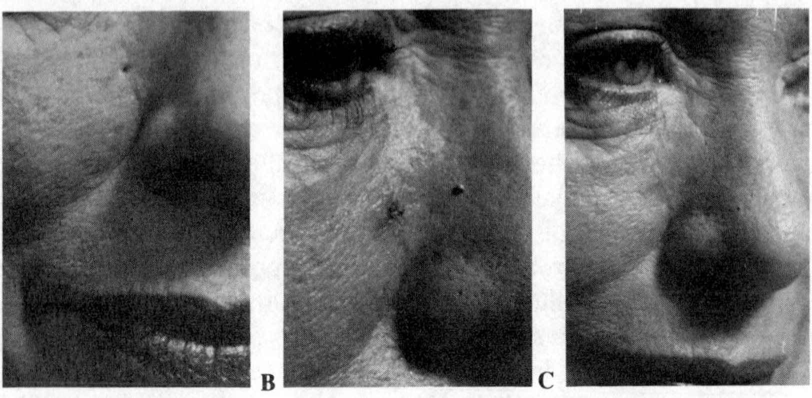

A B C

Figure 5-2 **A.** Deep pore not readily covered with makeup. **B.** Pore removed with minute punch, several fine sutures inserted. **C.** One month postoperative; fine scar practically invisible.

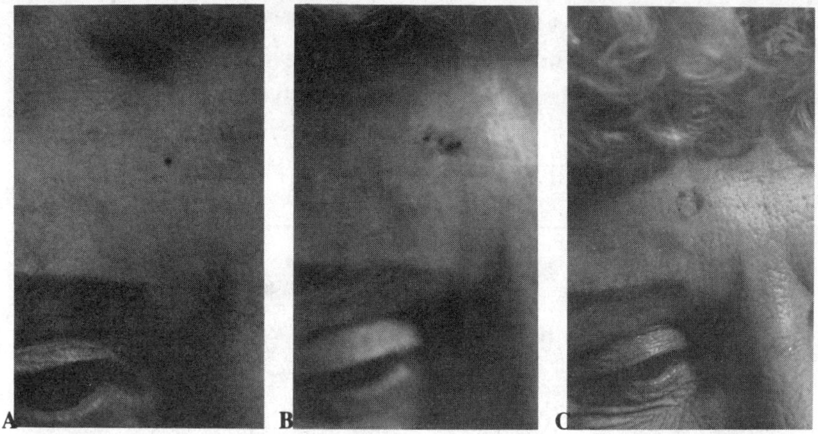

Figure 5-3 A. Deep pore of forehead. **B.** Fourth postoperative day. **C.** Eight days postoperative.

incision and drainage of the cysts and boils. The degree of improvement depends upon the nature of the scarring. Best results are obtained when there are shallow, well-defined pits. In contrast, poorly defined "ice-pick" scars yield less dramatically to abrasion. They, like large dilated pores, are often improved by removing them with a small (1–2 millimeter) circular punch while the skin is stretched perpendicular to the cutaneous lines of the face. This results in a tiny oval defect that easily converts to a line with its long axis in the same direction as the expression line of the skin. Several sutures maintain wound apposition and the healing yields an imperceptible scar where once a deep pore existed (Figures 5-2, 5-3).

How It's Done

Complete dermabrasion of the face is usually a hospital procedure, is performed under a general anesthetic and takes about an hour. The abrasion is carried out using a high-speed surgical planer equipped with an abrasive rotary wheel. After the sanding, the dermabraded skin is usually left exposed. The planed skin tends to ooze a yellowish serum that develops into a firm crust within twenty-four hours. Slight swelling and pain are normal reactions. Discomfort is easily remedied by analgesics. Most patients look worse than they feel. When the entire face is abraded, it is not unusual for the eyes to be swollen shut for several days. As the crust forms, the mouth is difficult to open, and most patients require a liquid diet for several days. The guaranteed weight loss is an added bonus of abrasion.

When the crust begins to crack, about the fourth or fifth day, itching or crawling sensations begin to signify healing. The crust is coated with antibiotic ointment on the fourth day and the patient is allowed to shower and shampoo his hair. From this moment

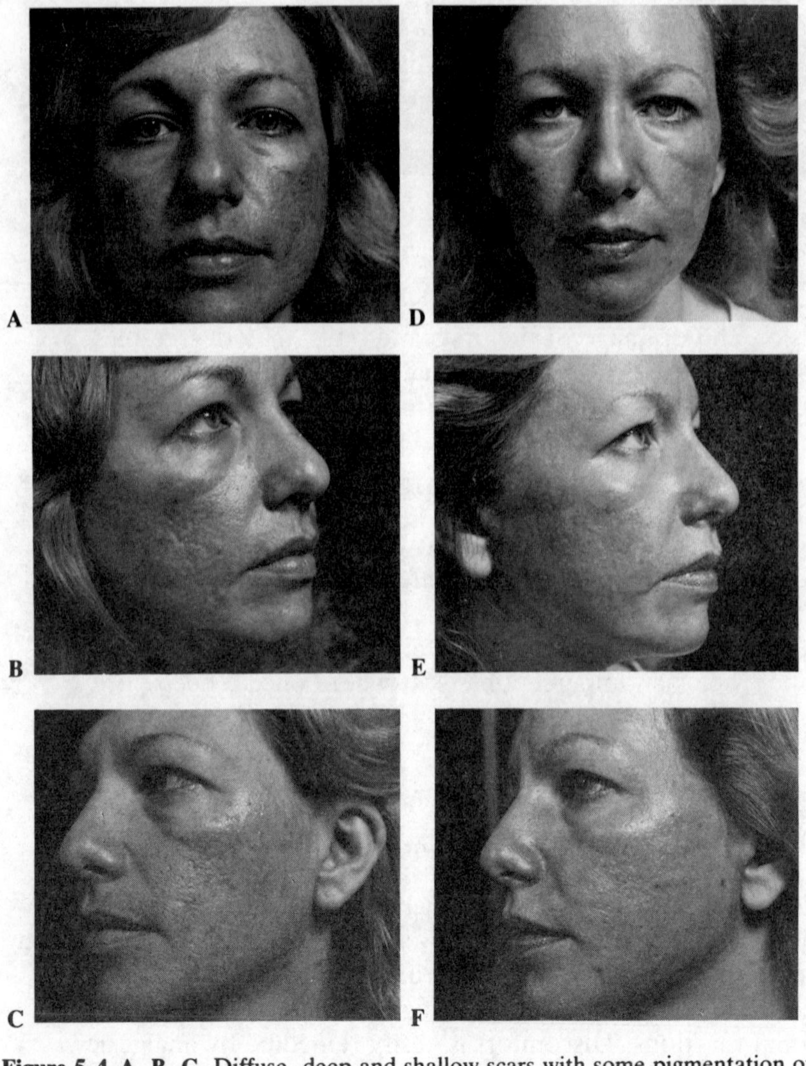

Figure 5-4 A, B, C. Diffuse, deep and shallow scars with some pigmentation of the face. **D, E, F.** Skin smoother, softer and lighter. Further abrasion will improve scars remaining—one-and-a-half months postoperative.

on, the crust will gradually strip off, revealing a pink and smoother skin. The initial appearance of the face is always superior to the final result since the swelling obscures any small scars that may still persist. The pinkness will remain for approximately four to six weeks, but may last for as long as three months (Figure 5-4).

Restrictions of routine activities are mainly social rather than arising from any physical discomfort. Limitations are largely self-imposed and depend on the degree of self-consciousness of the patient. If just a small portion of the face has been sanded and if the patient is not embarrassed by his appearance, he can return to work in several days following the procedure.

The skin remains tender for several weeks and is easily damaged by sunlight or minor trauma such as scratching. Therefore, it is essential to shield this new skin from sunlight until it has regained its normal tone; failure to do so can result in pigmentation changes that may take months to lose. For a similar period of time, the patient should also avoid vigorous facial scrubbing. Women may wear cosmetics by the third week, but men should postpone shaving until the crust has fallen off.

Postoperative office visits are infrequent as the patient renders the care necessary following dermabrasion or chemosurgery, with specific instructions from the surgeon.

To resurface the face by dermabrasion entails a surgical fee of $1500 to $2000; added to this cost is that of an anesthesiologist and a one-day hospital stay. Repeated planings are subject to a decreasing fee scale.

Peeling: Back to a Peach

The second fundamental procedure for improving the skin is chemosurgery or, as it is popularly known, peeling. Whereas dermabrasion mechanically removes the outer layers of the skin, chemosurgery performs the same process chemically. A face-lift can remove some deep wrinkles, but cannot alter the skin's quality or minimize the fine, intrinsic lines. Most acne and chicken-pox scars are deep whereas wrinkles and pigmentations are superficial. Therefore scars are handled with dermabrasion as this procedure can be employed deeper with more control and safety than can chemosurgery.

Particularly helped by peeling are the shallow and moderately deep facial wrinkles, freckles, pigmentations, and skin blemishes.

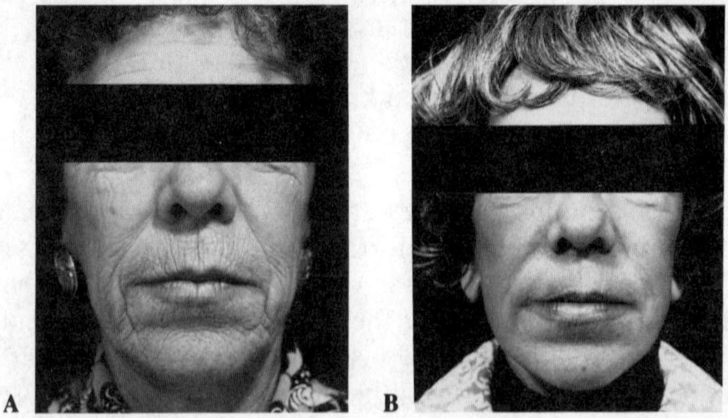

Figure 5-5 A. Deeply lined and wrinkled skin, probably genetic in origin. **B.** Seven months postpeel.

Eyelid wrinkles that might persist following blepharoplasty respond well to this method. The vertical lines around the mouth are almost completely eradicated by the peel.* The ideal patient is a fair-haired, fair-skinned, light-eyed person with "weather-beaten" skin. She is a peeling paradise for that tired and wrinkled face can be turned back into a smooth and velvety peach (Figure 5-5).

As with abrasion, peeling does not help either pores or the tiny capillaries that become noticeable with aging. In fact, both may be more conspicuous following the process.

The chemical agent most frequently used in peeling is a phenol compound that is applied either alone or with other chemicals to enhance or buffer its effect. One should be extremely selective and cautious in choosing an experienced and competent physician when considering this procedure, for harmful internal effects and facial scarring are more likely to occur at the hands of those having little or no training in this process.

It's the "Peel" That Rings Out the Old Face

Face peeling creates a more youthful appearance. Because there is an overall contraction following chemosurgery, there is a general tightening and retraction of the epidermal layer. The skin

**These lines occur much earlier in women than men because of men's thicker skin and more fat plus the stabilizing effect of the large and abundant hair follicles that are present in men.*

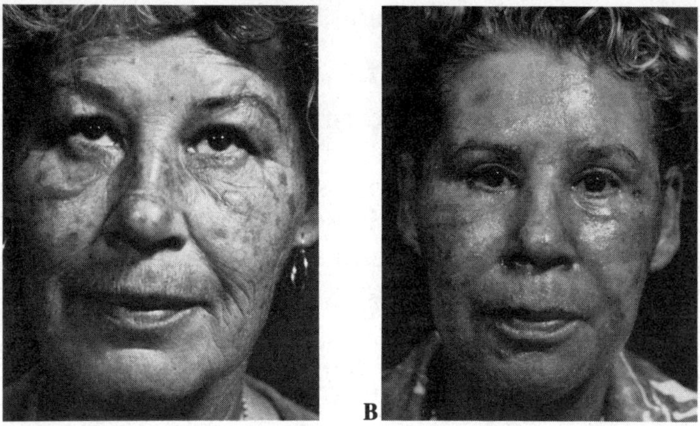

A B

Figure 5-6 **A.** Numerous facial pigmentations together with wrinkles. **B.** Ten days postpeel; same patient as in Figure 3-8.

appears firmer, smoother, and more elastic. Its texture becomes softer and the complexion brighter (Figure 5-6).

The prevention of complications is contingent upon excluding certain patients and recognizing the kind of skin that is to be treated. Phenols are nephropathic agents and are capable of aggravating or even producing kidney damage. Since phenols are detoxified by the liver, the functional integrity of the liver should be ascertained before the procedure. No one with a history of liver or kidney disease should undergo chemosurgery using phenols as the cauterant. Diabetics (whether controlled or not), those with a tendency to form keloids, or anyone in poor nutritional status that could delay or complicate the healing process *should never* be peeled with *any* type of cauterant.

The face should never be peeled at the same time a face-lift is performed, not even small portions such as the lips, chin, or forehead. The swelling that occurs with surgery can extend to these areas and impair the local blood supply thereby jeopardizing healing of the burned regions and possibly leading to the formation of scars. A full face-peel may be performed approximately six to eight weeks after surgery and spot peels are safe about one week from the day of the operation.

Because face peeling is uncomfortable, both physically and psychologically, the procedure is better tolerated if performed in a hospital. However, with proper sedation and intravenous tranquilizers, many patients can safely undergo chemosurgery in the surgeon's office with only minor discomfort.

How It's Done

Preoperative preparations for chemosurgery are similar to those for an abrasion except for one added step; the oil from the face is removed with ether or acetone to ensure uniform penetration of the phenol solution. No anesthesia is required, as in dermabrasion. Only sedation, which suspends the stinging, combined with intravenous Valium®, which produces amnesia for the procedure, is used.

Upon contact with phenol, the skin immediately blanches to a frosty-white color, then changes to a dark red tone several minutes later (Figure 5-7). In essence, it is receiving a superficial second-degree burn. Initially the patient experiences a burning sensation that, in most cases, subsides after five or ten minutes. Although the entire painting process could be performed in approximately ten minutes or so, the face is treated slowly in sections (approximately one hour) to minimize rapid absorption by the skin and possible danger to the liver and kidneys. The peel is carried under the jaw line so that any demarcation between the neck and face is well hidden by the shadow of the jaw.

Following the painting process, the face is covered with multiple strips of tape, leaving only the eyes, nostrils, and lips exposed (Figure 5-8). Taping prevents evaporation and drying of

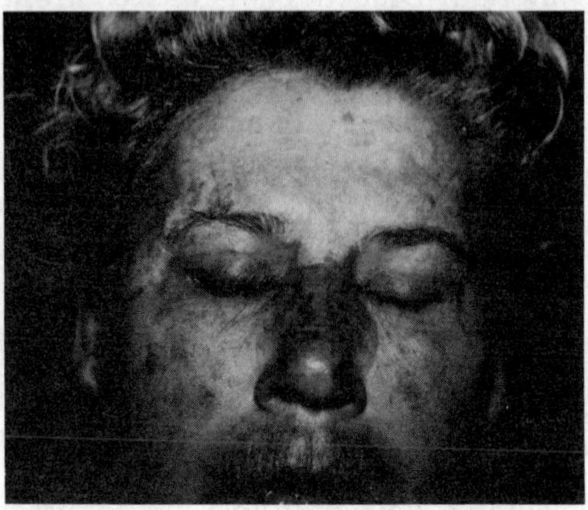

Figure 5-7 Peeled skin frosts immediately upon contact with acid.

the serum that exudes from the irritated skin, and thus heightens skin maceration. The procedure thus renders a deeper peel, and is recommended for the severely weather-beaten face. Without taping, little maceration of the face occurs. The open method produces surface skin peeling and is indicated for less harshly aged skin. This surface peel chiefly rids the face of freckles, pigmentations, blemishes, and fine wrinkles, and is designed mainly to give the face a cleaner and fresher look.

With the face taped, there is considerable swelling and discomfort during the first day; however, prescribed analgesics control any severe or throbbing pain. Within twenty-four to forty-eight hours the tape is removed, not a painful step since the

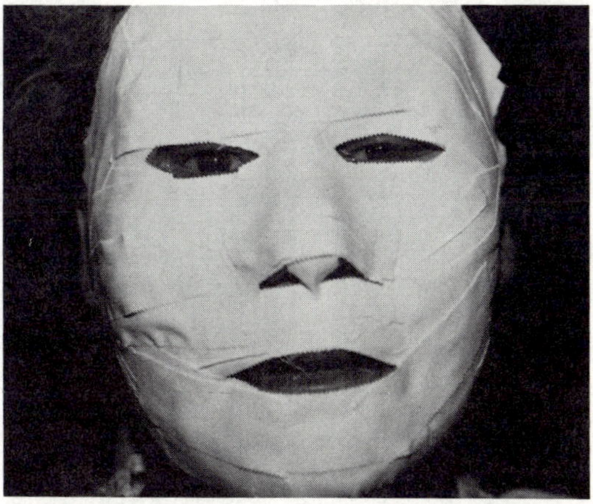

Figure 5-8 Immediately following the peel, the face is taped to heighten the reaction.

exuded serum has loosened the tape. The macerated skin is sprinkled with an antiseptic powder to form a protective crust. From this point on, discomfort will be minimal. This powdering is repeated by the patient over the next few days until a brown granular mask develops. On the fourth day after the peel, ointment is liberally applied to the mask to soften it, and the patient is instructed to shower and shampoo her hair. As in abrasion, the mask strips away shortly thereafter.

Considerable swelling of the face, neck, and eyelids persists for the first three or four days. As it is difficult to open the mouth, liquids or a soft diet are the nutritional mainstays. Oral hygiene can be accomplished with a dental pick or mouth washes. Without taping (open method), both swelling and discomfort are less and the entire process is more easily tolerated. With either method, the face will shed the crust, or mask, approximately five to six days from the phenol application. The relief that the patient experiences as this crust sloughs off is only rivaled by the stunning appearance of the face.* The new skin will be pink, smoother, softer, and more resilient to the touch. The reupholstering, in a sense, has replaced leather with velvet (Figure 5-9).

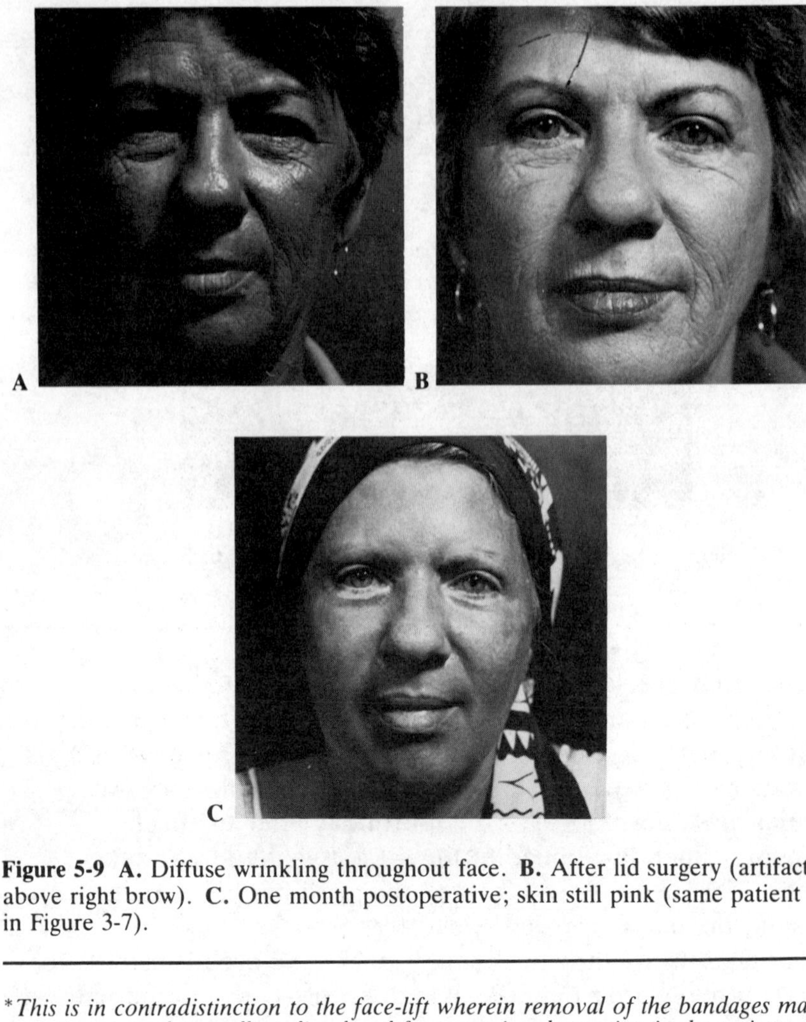

Figure 5-9 **A.** Diffuse wrinkling throughout face. **B.** After lid surgery (artifact above right brow). **C.** One month postoperative; skin still pink (same patient as in Figure 3-7).

**This is in contradistinction to the face-lift wherein removal of the bandages may sometimes reveal a swollen, discolored face, causing depression in the patient.*

Persistent swelling may hide residual wrinkles. As this puffiness decreases, some lines may return and patients should be forewarned of this to avoid disappointment. The pink tone of the face gradually fades over the next three months.

Once the mask has fallen away, the patient may wash her face with soap and water. Her skin may be quite dry and she can use any emollient to soften it. She may resume using cosmetics one week after the mask has been removed. She should rigidly avoid exposure to sunlight for at least three months—irregular pigmentation is the probable penalty if this advice is not heeded. If pigmentary changes do occur, they can be lightened by bleaching creams or, at a later date, by using a lighter peel solution without taping.

A serious but infrequent complication of chemosurgery is scarring. The incidence is higher on the chin and neck, but can occur in any area where the caustic has been applied. There also may be a slight coarsening of the skin texture, exhibiting an orange peel effect. Not every face requires taping. If the skin is thick, leathery, and sun-baked, taping should and can be performed with minimum risk. Thin, fine-textured skin with shallow lines and wrinkling can be improved without any occlusive dressing. Taping enhances skin maceration, causing increased surface damage, which carries the risk of increased phenol penetration and dermal scarring.*

How long will the benefits of a peel last? Again, it depends on the patient's living pattern. Five or ten years after the procedure, the patient will certainly reflect a more youthful look than if she had never undergone chemosurgery. The less sun exposure she gets from the time of the peel on, the less wrinkled and more youthful she will appear. If necessary, chemosurgery can be performed again since skin regenerates to about 90 percent of its previous thickness following the procedure.

Meet Beverly

This case history demonstrates the remarkable benefits of chemosurgery: Bev was a forty-two-year-old woman who requested a face-peel. Throughout her youth she had sunned herself at resorts from Europe to Mexico. As she grew older, the

**Following chemosurgery, the epidermis sheds, and a new, smooother epidermis appears. However, the epidermis is only a thin, cellular layer about as thick as the sheet of paper you are now reading. It is in the thicker dermis that the most meaningful changes take place, and it is here where great scarring can occur.*

effects of following the sun had caught up with her.

She had been divorced for some time and her spousal support had run out. She was forced to seek employment to sustain any semblance of her usual life-style. Obtaining work was not that easy, and she felt that her appearance was the chief obstacle in securing a decent position for she had to compete with many talented and younger-looking people.

"I've always felt that my face was so white and pasty without a tan. Hell, in my circle of friends we were practically graded on our tans. Well, I know now that I could have added rouge and color and removed that pale look. Now I have lines that I can't rub away. When I look into the mirror, it's hard for me to believe that I once was a cute baby. It's even difficult to have dates. Men don't see my character or virtues. They are more interested in looking at the landscape."

With just casual inspection, the view was not what you would call handsome. Her face had become traitor to her body for although she still had a superbly sculpted figure, her skin was grooved with a maze of backroads that meandered aimlessly over her features. Her silky, aggressive manner belied her appearance; here sat an imposter for emotionally she was a young woman held hostage inside an old wrinkled face.

Chemosurgery was discussed with her. It was explained that since she was so deeply lined, taping would be required. She was terribly apprehensive as she had heard many horrible tales of the firelike pain and possible scarring that could occur when the face was peeled. Her fear was overcome by her desire, and the procedure was planned for the hospital.

Although her sedation was quite deep she was so nervous that a light general anesthetic was required for the process. This kept her in a deeply sedated state with no discomfort throughout the day. The next day the tape removal and antiseptic powdering were uneventful. Her prunelike skin slid off with the mask five days later. Although red and puffed, she was unrecognizable from her former self. Within three weeks, she was back in circulation, and within two months she had procured a position as a buyer in a high-fashion woman's shop. Not only was she employed, but a man she cared for had become seriously interested in her as well. She was happy, even ecstatic, as she spoke of her new situation: "Life is so different since my peel. Before it was so empty. Now I have something to do, someone to love, and something to look forward to."

Refurbishing the face with a peel costs approximately $1000 without taping and about $2000 with taping as those who are taped require greater time and care. Collagen, silicone, or fibrin-foam injections range from $50 to $200 per session. In some instances, dermabrasion is covered by insurance. The other treatments are not.

Zap, Crackle and Frost

Electrosurgery is the modality used for removing warts, other superficial growths, and capillaries. These defects all become more noticeable with age. The epidermis thins and the elastic fibers encircling the blood vessels weaken and rupture, spilling blood into the surrounding skin. As the skin's biochemistry changes, degenerative changes take place, yielding a variety of benign and malignant growths such as cysts, warts, keratoses, and cancers.

By the use of a minimal electric current through a fine needle, many of these lesions can be burned flat and the blood vessels coagulated. Healing is rapid with little scarring.

Another less widely known process for removing superficial growths is the application of liquid nitrogen. Whereas electrosurgery eliminates these by coagulation of the tissue through heat, the application of liquid nitrogen accomplishes the same purpose by intense cold. The reaction of the skin to freezing is less and a better scar can result. Pain and bleeding are also not so severe with this technique. However, it cannot be used for fine vessels or capillaries.

Small veins and sunburst capillaries, long the bane of women's faces and legs, can be corrected by a procedure known as compression sclerotherapy. With this method, using an extremely small needle and under high-powered magnification, a minute amount of a diluted sclerosing agent is injected into these tiny vessels. No anesthetic is required as the small, sharp needle thrust is virtually painless. The sclerosing solution produces an irritation of the vein or capillary and in so doing obliterates it. Mild compression of the area is performed for several minutes and then the patient can go about her daily routine. After several treatments, the veins or capillaries are eradicated. However, as this is a progressive disease, further treatments may be needed in a few years' time.

The Thin Red Line

All surgeries begin with an incision and end with a scar. The

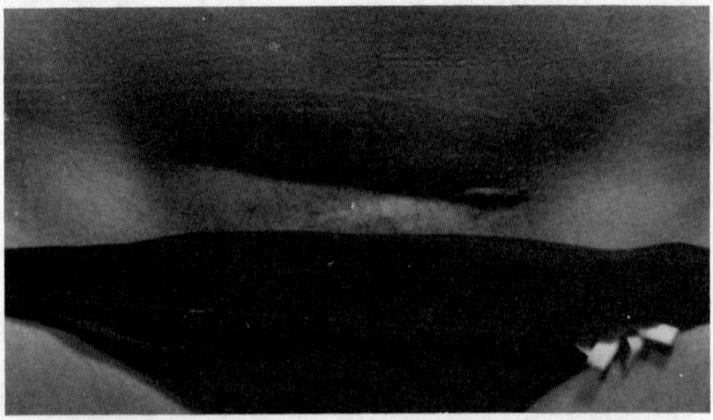

A

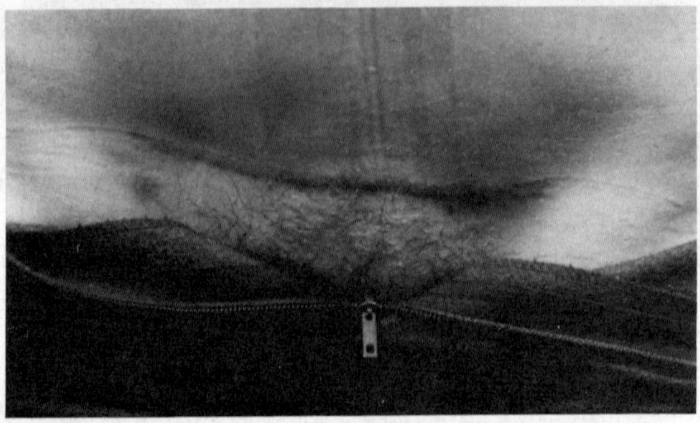

B

Figure 5-10 A. Keloid following laparatomy; itching and pain were the symptoms. **B.** One month postoperative. Although the scar is somewhat longer, it is less obvious. With added time, the scar will blend in more and become imperceptible.

final resolution of any incision, any laceration, any cut, is a scar. Yet the placement and closure of skin incisions form one of the most neglected aspects of general surgery. In many instances, it is the sole criterion, the ultimate trademark, by which a patient appraises the competence of a surgeon—the finer the scar, the better the surgeon. In the course of an injury, not only is the skin often cut, but failing adequate correction of the wound, the psyche is also lacerated. Minimizing the visible scar following an operation constitutes one of the major goals of the cosmetic surgeon.

Scars are least conspicuous and best camouflaged when placed within a wrinkle, a contour line, or the hair. Eyelid incisions leave imperceptible scars as do incisions on the palms and soles.

In certain areas of the body associated with movement—shoulders, chest, knees, elbows, and hips—scars are very evident, even though primary closure leaves a fine scar. The constant movement, twist, torque, and tension placed on these scars inevitably cause them to spread. The chest and back are particularly notorious for poor healing, and in these areas a keloid, an exuberant and abnormal type of scarring, may occur (Figure 5-10).

Massaging the scar with vitamin E, aloe vera extract, cocoa butter or other creams, has been proposed to soften and minimize a scar. While these substances do no harm, the benefit accrued is really due to the massage alone, which by itself tends to soften the scar. The massage benefits the patient psychologically as he becomes involved and is contributing to his own healing. Since most scars improve spontaneously, tincture of time is the best medicine. Time is a lousy beautician, but a great healer.

"Beauty is only skin deep" is the standard cliché that is literally so true, for if this ornamental blanket that envelops us from head to toe were shaved to a depth of several millimeters, we would all look much the same. But it is no cliché that all true beauty begins with beautiful skin. The female of the species is generally more sensitive to her facial appearance than the male. She is, by tradition, cast into the role of the pursued. Advertisements, sponsored by the cosmetic industry, insist that a flawless skin will ensure that pursuit. Creams, lotions, and gels can lubricate the skin, and cosmetics can conceal a multitude of faults. But surgery has the greatest appeal, for only peeling and planing have a long-standing effect and yield the smoothest of skins.

Q&A

Is it risky to have silicone injected in your face and is it safe to use?

Risk is an inevitable fact of life and implicit in our lives at all times. By contrast, what is meant by safe? What we have learned of this controversial substance over a twenty-year period is that when properly used, it is effective and safe for most people. There will always be those who will react adversely to any drug or substance and for them, the risk will be greater and the therapy not as safe.

Which is better for lines and wrinkles, dermabrasion or peeling?

Both will rid the face of most lines, wrinkles, and pigmentations. However, the peeling process chemically rearranges the collagen fibers within the dermis and literally creates a newer and younger skin. Thus the effects of peeling last much longer than sanding (dermabrasion).

What's the best treatment for my acne scars?

Since scars are deeper than wrinkles, dermabrasion is safer to use than peeling. If the acid goes too deep, further scarring will result. Most surgeons know how to control their hands when using the abrader and can readily guide the sanding to the proper level.

How can I get rid of the tiny blood vessels in my face?

These can be eradicated by inserting a tiny thin wire into the vessel and delivering a small current through it, causing the vessel to blanch out. The procedure is tedious and may require repeating, but eventually the vessels will disappear.

Prevention is better than treatment. Avoid all heat to the face. Therefore, wash your face with cool to tepid water. Avoid saunas and all stimulating drinks such as tea or coffee. Candlelight and wine may sound romantic, but you will be better off if you keep the candlelight and throw away the wine. All alcoholic beverages cause vasodilation that encourage the reappearance of these capillaries.

What is the best treatment for acne?

This dermatological condition is so variable from patient to patient that no one explicit treatment can be given that will work for everyone. Basically, you should be under a physician's care and should follow his advice. Never attack the face. Do not squeeze or pick the pimples for this can lead to further infection and scarring. Screen out foods that you have learned will cause facial eruptions and make every effort to keep both your hair and face as clean as possible.

6

Tresses and Locks—Gone Today, Hair Tomorrow

Hair is an offshoot of the skin. Biologically inert, it isn't essential. But its absence or overabundance in certain parts of the body can engender anxiety in both sexes. For a man's face value drops with falling hair and a woman's sexual value decreases as hair proliferates on her facial skin. Psychologists might well investigate our compelling interest in it for although an inactive substance, hair generates a brisk business.

Where There's Hair . . .

The initial function of human hair was as protection against physical injury, insulation against the cold and a warning device against insects. As man evolved into a hunter and developed speed for running, a means was needed for ridding the body of heat produced during the chase. Elimination of body hair and the development of sweat glands were evolution's response. As people learned to clothe themselves and build shelters, the need for hair as insulation was further reduced. Hair has still retained its tactile function as a warning device against insects, but in our mechanized world, it offers scant protection against trauma.

Where and What It's Like

Most parts of the body except the palms and soles have hair follicles and hair that emerges from certain parts still retains a function. The brows inhibit sweat from dripping into the eyes and the lashes act as dust catchers, as do the hairs in the nose and ears. Armpit hair facilitates the swinging of the arms and pubic hair prevents chafing during sex. But for the most part, evolution has consigned hair to merely an ornamental role, although it has deep sexual and psychological roots.

Like skin, hair color is determined genetically and, except by chemical means, cannot be changed. Whether hair glimmers like wheat or smoulders like slate depends upon the amount of pigment (melanin) within the body. Hair loses its color and whitens as pigment production decreases. "Salt and pepper" hair as an entity does not exist—the white hairs scattered throughout the more numerous brown or black ones give the illusion of gray hair. Although premature grayness can occur in the twenties or thirties, most people experience graying in their forties. It usually begins at the temples and gradually extends to the front and center; the back of the head is the last place to lose color. Eyebrows can whiten with age, although they lose pigmentation less rapidly than scalp hair. Except in rare instances, eyelashes preserve their pigmentation and do not become gray with age.

Hair can be grouped by hormonal classification into two types. Eyelashes, brows, and hair on the limbs and fingers are independent of sex hormones, and are influenced by the growth hormone secreted by the small pituitary gland located deep within the brain. Beards; moustaches; pubic, axillary, nasal, and ear hair; and most body, arm, and leg hair are under the control of the sex hormones. Both the sex and growth hormones regulate scalp hair; the male hormone gives rise to excessive hair loss in both sexes when the individuals are genetically programmed in that fashion.

The average scalp containing brunette hair (which is thickest) has slightly more than 100,000 hairs; blondes, who have the finest hair, have a greater number and redheads fewer. The eyebrows contain about 600 hairs and the eyelashes of both lids have approximately 150. A woman's hair is usually thicker than a man's. Examination of a hair under a microscope reveals that a straight hair is round, wavy hair is oval, and curly or kinky hair is flat or kidney-shaped.

When hair first emerges from the scalp, it grows at a rate of a half inch per month. Cutting or shaving the hair has no effect on its growth rate; short hair seems to grow faster because, over any brief time interval, its percentage increase is greater. Women grow scalp hair faster than men. Between fifteen and thirty years of age, hair undergoes its fastest growth. At about fifty or sixty years, activity declines and growth is minimal beyond sixty-five. Greater growth occurs in the spring and summer months than at other times of the year.

How It Does and Doesn't Grow

Hairs are continually being shed as others are growing.

Approximately 100 hairs are lost daily from the scalp. As long as the rate of regrowth keeps pace with the fallout rate, the person maintains a full head of hair. When regrowth lags or when the follicles become diseased or are destroyed, thinning or baldness occurs. The hair-cycle disruptions are reversible when disease occurs and if the pathologic cause is removed.

Pattern disturbances, on the other hand, are generally irreversible and over 95 percent of all hair loss is due to this. Male-pattern-baldness is unrelated to poor scalp circulation, dandruff, the wearing or non-wearing of hats or the innumerable other myths. Male-pattern-baldness is not the result of a skin disease, but comes from the shrinking and withering of individual hair follicles that cause them to perish before their master does. Since there are no known drugs, remedies, or external devices that will replace hair follicles, this type of baldness is considered permanent and incurable.

By all scientific evidence, male-pattern-baldness is a genetically transferred, hormone-dependent condition. Sex, age, and heredity are the three factors involved and there isn't much we can do about any one of them. Inheritance of the balding propensity is a complex phenomenon; the genes can be transmitted through either the male or the female line, although it is not exceptional for the succession to pass over one or more generations. Essentially, balding in men is genetically dominant (inheritable from either one or both parents); in women, it constitutes a limited recessive type as both parents must transmit the balding-prone gene to produce hair loss.

Male hormones are the second factor and predominantly trigger male-pattern-baldness. It matters not how great the inherited tendency; baldness of this type cannot surface without the male hormone, nor can this hormone induce baldness if one is not genetically prone. Regardless of hereditary tendency, eunuchs never develop male-pattern-baldness; men castrated after this type of baldness has begun demonstrate no further hair loss. This form of treatment, to date, has not been greeted with immense enthusiasm by the average male.

Simply growing old constitutes the third component of baldness. Some loss of hair with age is universal; it is the rare seventy-year-old who retains all his hair of his twenties. Even though the amount of male hormone decreases with age, this small amount is enough to perpetuate balding.

This type of baldness has a characteristic pattern and course and progresses slowly over several years. It begins with a gradual recession of the hairline at the temples, and eventually the frontal hairline forms the shape of the letter **M** (the widow's peak). Soon the hair at the crown becomes thin and the sparseness advances toward the forehead. As the bare areas merge with time, only a horseshoe fringe remains. This fringe is rarely affected in male-pattern-baldness; it is the mother-lode for hair transplantation.

If the pattern-baldness occurs shortly after adolescence, the prognosis is poor as these individuals are likely to be quite bald before their thirtieth birthday. If one has not lost half his hair by age thirty, it is unlikely that he will ever be extremely bald. Because baldness in women rarely shows a steadily receding hairline (thinning is more likely), it is not generally recognized that women also suffer from pattern-baldness.

There are other forms of baldness—those from illness, stress, emotional upsets, and the like. For the most part, these are temporary and it is among sufferers from these types that unscrupulous hair restorers find their most gullible clientele. The so-called hair and scalp specialist often uses before-and-after pictures of persons who have had one of the temporary forms of baldness as a gimmick to attract customers and to attest to their own effectiveness. The deception lies in the fact that in such case regrowth would have occurred without treatment.

The Cover-Up

Wigs, Weaves, and Implants

Easily the safest and most effective way of cosmetically covering a bald head is with a hairpiece (Figure 6-1). However, toupees are hot and uncomfortable in warm climates and are expensive as well ($800 to $1500). They also require, at additional cost, constant care and must be replaced every two to three years, depending on care, cleaning, and type of hair used (most hairpieces have 20 percent human and 80 percent synthetic hair). Synthetic hair is preferable because the color doesn't fade as rapidly nor does it tangle as easily as human hair.

Another method used to cover balding is hair-weaving. This is a nonsurgical procedure wherein a nonshrinking nylon thread is woven and braided into the horseshoe fringe of hair on the patient's head. A matching hairpiece with an interwoven base is then sewn onto these nylon threads. After shampooing, cutting, and styling, the result is a hairpiece attached to a nylon-thread

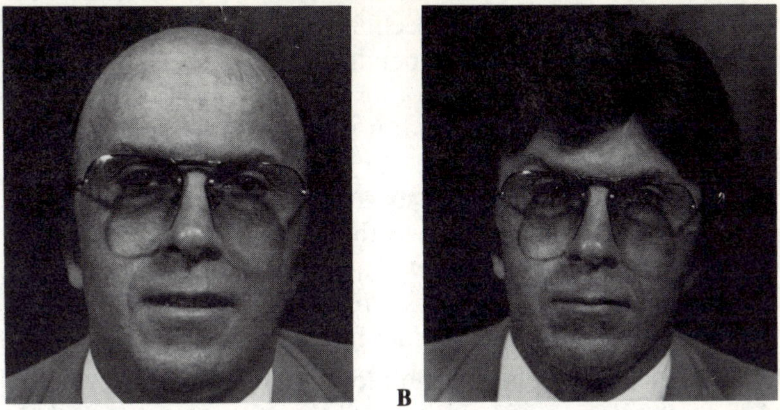

A B

Figure 6-1 A hairpiece makes the wearer younger and more attractive. In fact, whenever the bald head is covered by anything such as a cap, hat, or turban, the wearer always appears younger. (Photos courtesy of Herb Yerman Esquire, Beverly Hills, CA.)

which is anchored to the patient's own hair. This technique overcomes the wearer's nagging fear of becoming unglued for it uses no glue or tape. It allows the wearer to swim, shower, or take part in active sports without fear of exposure. However, it also has its drawbacks.

The entire process requires two to three hours at a minimum cost of $900 to $1200. Because the attached hair grows, gradually moving away from the scalp, the hairpiece becomes more and more loose over the scalp. The nylon thread must be reanchored and adjusted lower along the hair shaft in pace with the growth. This maintenance is required every four to six weeks depending on the rate of growth; each session costs approximately $50. It is very difficult for the patient to clean properly beneath the net-like base and this can cause annoying odors. And the hair to which the hairpiece is attached can, with time, be lost as a result of traction, leading to worsening of the client's baldness.

The implantation of hair fiber was once quite fashionable. The hair was imbedded into a firm fiber strut much like the eyelet of a shoelace. The solid ends were then implanted into the scalp and did create a luxurious head of hair. Unfortunately, they also caused a marked foreign-body reaction, resulting in infection, pain, and scarring. This method is mentioned for historical interest only; it is not recommended.

Surgical Treatment

In the late 1950s the surgical technique of hair transplantation was introduced. This method depends on the established fact that hair moved from one area to another on the scalp will behave and grow with the same vigor that it did in its original location. This technique does not increase the number of hairs on the head; it merely redistributes the existing hair. Transplanting hair plugs from one part of the scalp to the needy part is the safest and most effective way of cosmetically covering a bald head via a surgical procedure. The surgical simplicity for the patient and ensuing minor discomfort are prime factors in its appeal.

The number of transplants required to give satisfactory results depends on the degree of baldness and the amount of donor hair that exists. (Approximately 60 to 80 percent of the hair in the horseshoe fringe can be removed without leaving noticeable gaps.) As few as forty or fifty transplants may be indicated for filling in a **V** or a slight recession at the temple, while it will take as many as 500 or more for relatively complete coverage of extensive baldness. A reasonable rate of transplantation is from forty to sixty plugs per session; quite often more are performed, but this may produce marked swelling and more discomfort for the patient.

The ideal patient is one who is curly-haired as this type of hair best hides any tell-tale scars. The ideal area of the scalp is the crown because this region can be easily filled in with virtually no evidence that the patient has had hair transplants. Establishing a new hairline presents more of a problem since the scars are usually visible, especially if the hair is combed back. To conceal this the patient will need to restyle his hair. In fact, any person contemplating hair transplants must be conscious of hairstyling to camouflage the scarring and tufting appearance that may result with this procedure.

Hair transplantation is an office procedure performed under a local analgesic and takes about one and a half hours. The patient need only shampoo his hair the day preceding the surgery. Usually the patient is sedated shortly after arriving at the doctor's office and is then placed in a semireclining position with his head elevated on a pillow or headrest. The hair of the donor site at the back of the head is trimmed, just enough hair being left to determine its slope. Determining the slope or direction of hair growth allows the surgeon to properly guide the instrument when removing donor plugs and prevents the accidental severing of hair roots. The recipient sites and donor areas are then cleansed and injected with the local.

Using a punch device (much like a cookie cutter that is less than a quarter inch in diameter), hair-bearing plugs of skin are bored out from the back and placed in a sterile salt solution as they are removed. The number of hairs appearing in each plug varies from person to person, usually ranging from six to fifteen. Next, the transplanter turns to the bald area and, with a slightly smaller punch, removes an equivalent number of prepatterned plugs of identical depth. Since these holes expand whereas the donor hair plugs contract, a snug fit is obtained. Whatever bleeding occurs is easily controlled by pressure. While the bald area is being made ready to receive the hair, the assistant trims any excess fat that might linger on the hair plugs. These fashioned hair plugs are then inserted into the openings in the bald area and pressed into place. No sutures are required as the fibrin blood clot literally glues the grafts into place. The donor areas are either sutured if a small number of plugs has been removed or, if a great number is taken, they are allowed to heal naturally. (The reason for the difference in treatment will be clear later in this chapter.) Both bald and donor areas are protected with gauze dressings and the head is bandaged. The patient is able to leave the office under his own power and drive home.

The physician removes the bandage after twenty-four hours and cleanses the scalp of dried blood. Over the next several days the grafts become encrusted. This crust separates in about ten to fourteen days leaving a pink circle of scar, whose coloring fades and disappears over the next several months. Donor sites heal in about two weeks. The scars in these areas shrink, lose their redness, and become pale in two or three months. As they are covered by the surrounding hair, they are invisible to ordinary scrutiny.

The original hair stubs in the grafts do not grow, but fall out within a month following the procedure. After an initial resting period of about ten to twelve weeks, a new generation of hair will appear at the surface of the scalp. This will retain the color and the general texture of the hair from the donor site. Quite often, however, the transplanted hair will grow out coarser and curlier than it was in the donor area. At present, there is no explanation for this in every case.* These transplanted hairs will follow their previous growth patterns and life cycles and, with careful technique, the "take" will approach 99 percent.

After completion of the operation, the patient can return to work the next day and may resume all normal, nonstrenuous activities; strenuous ones have to wait for ten days. Since few people work on Saturday, a favorite day for transplantation is Friday. When Monday rolls around, there is minimal evidence of the procedure. As the grafts should be left undisturbed for the first two weeks, combing or brushing is not allowed in the surgical sites. The patient may shampoo his hair on the fourth day after transplantation. The grafts itch with healing and the physician will prescribe a soothing salve to minimize this. Picking or scratching the grafts could cause bleeding or infection. A hairpiece can be worn within a few days following the surgery. For those who do not wear toupees, the grafts can be cloaked by restyling the remaining hair over and around them.

An entire bald head is not filled in at one sitting as hair transplants cannot be placed one next to the other without interrupting the circulation, and thus creating the probability of a poor take. It requires at least four sessions to fill one given area solidly (Figure 6-2). The intervals between these sessions vary

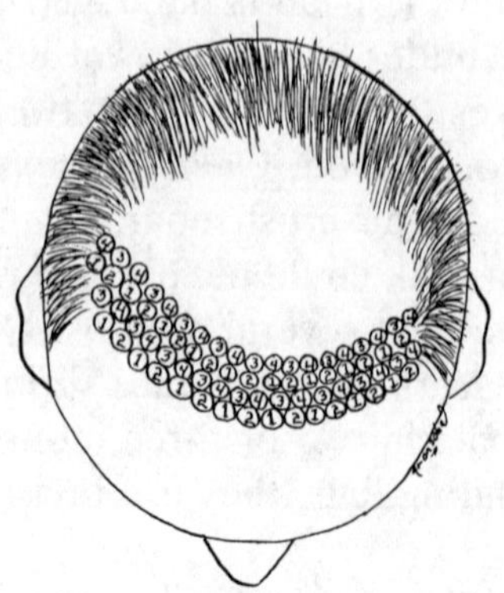

Figure 6-2 Four separate sessions usually complete a given area of the scalp. The third and fourth sessions are performed three months respectively after sessions one and two. Subsequently, 2-3 mm hair grafts may be required to fill in the small gaps between the large grafts to produce a thicker density.

**Stuffing a donor plug into a recipient site of inadequate depth can squash the hair follicle and cause curly hair growth where hair was straight in the donor plug. An inadequate depth at the recipient site can also result in the elevation of the plug that yields a cobblestone feel and appearance at the recipient site.*

from surgeon to surgeon. Transplantation appears to be most successful when the second session is approximately four to six weeks after the first and the subsequent sessions are delayed until hair has begun growing from the first two transplants. The last transplantation should not be performed until growth has started from the third. When the hair in transplanted plugs begins to grow, the surgeon can more accurately ascertain where to place future plugs so the hair growth will appear more natural instead of like so many tufts growing out from the scalp.

Some Vexing Considerations

Infections from the transplanting process are rare, but antibiotics are routinely prescribed for prophylactic measures. Although it is unlikely that the patient will need them, physicians routinely prescribe a small supply of an analgesic medication. Occasionally some painless and harmless swelling develops along the forehead and eyelids but this disappears within several days. Numbness and tingling sensations may occur during the course of the treatment; they are temporary and disappear within a few months as the nerve endings regrow.

As mentioned, occasionally there may be a change of texture as the new hair grows out. Other disadvantages of the punch graft technique are the possible "honeycomb scarring" pattern that may occur in the recipient area, the "buckshot" appearance of the donor sites when numerous plugs have been removed, and a cobblestone feel at the recipient site. When a limited number of grafts (thirty to fifty) are taken at each session, the donor punches can be arranged so that they can be closed with absorbable sutures, leaving a fine scar that is rarely visible. When many grafts are taken, it is impossible to suture the punched out donor areas without distorting the surrounding tissue. These openings each leave a circular bald area that is more noticeable. Taking fewer grafts at each session does prolong the process, but also ensures less swelling and discomfort as well as minimal scarring.

Another disadvantage of hair transplants is that it is difficult to obtain a thick hair density. It is also impossible to cover large areas of baldness completely. The patient must be satisfied with only partial coverage of his scalp. The prolonged course of multiple procedures and the cost ($1000 to $8000) may also be deterrents (approximately $15 to $25 per hair plug). Because hair circulation is interrupted, the follicles go into a resting phase wherein the old hair falls out and the new doesn't reappear for approximately three months. Since new growth requires several months and a cosmetically significant growth may take as long as six months to a year, the procedure extends over a long time. Only patients who are highly motivated and have a realistic attitude as to what can be accomplished should undertake hair transplantation.

And last but not least, the patient should be aware that further natural hair loss may occur, with the possibility of continuing baldness. The transplanted hairs, however, will survive to the full extent of their donor area life-potential, and may appear isolated as other hair in their new neighborhood disappears.

For men with a large area of baldness, the cosmetic results of hair transplantation may be somewhat disappointing. Yet thinning hair and baldness in men are not a trivial condition—the billion-dollar annual sales of hair products attest to that fact. Even

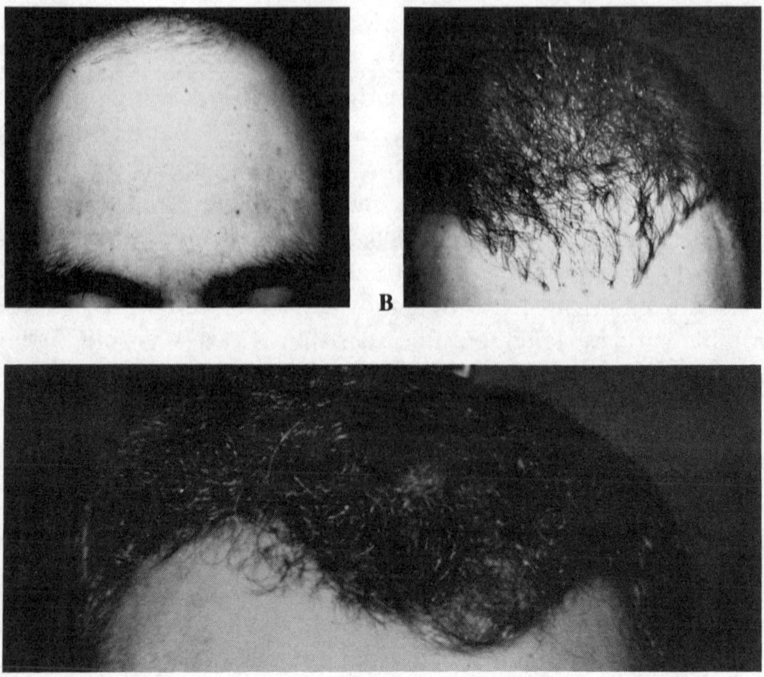

A B C

Figure 6-3 A. A 22-year-old with thinning and balding hair. **B.** Eight months later after seventy hair plants. **C.** Two years after first photo following a total of 220 hair transplants. (Photos courtesy of Jerome Kirschbaum, MD, San Francisco, CA.)

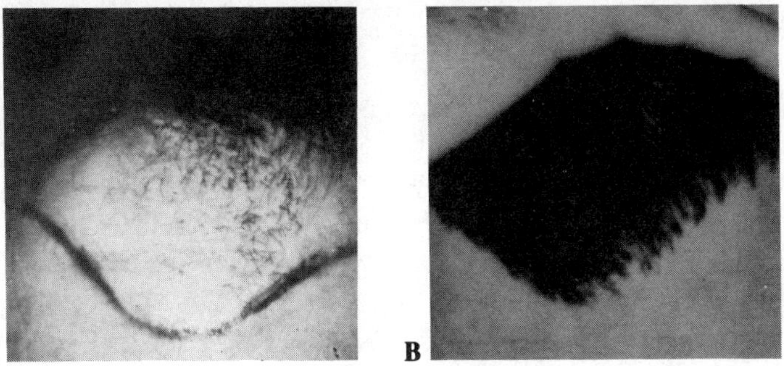

A B

Figure 6-4 A. A 44-year-old man with marked frontal recession. **B.** Ten months later after 320 hair transplants; will require some 2 mm plugs to give a fuller, more natural hairline. (Photos courtesy of Konstantine Sparkuhl, MD, Newport, CA.)

modest improvement has been shown to create new images and strengthen shaky egos. Typical changes in appearance achieved in hair transplantation are illustrated in Figures 6-3, 4, 5.

How this improvement can change one's life-style is shown in the following case history: David was a young physician who began to experience severe hair loss at nineteen years. He had tried without success all the advertised remedies to prevent further loss. By his late twenties his entire crown was bald; all that remained was a horseshoe fringe of hair.

"I spend too much time thinking about my baldness and I know that I would feel insecure and tense with a toupee. I'm tired of

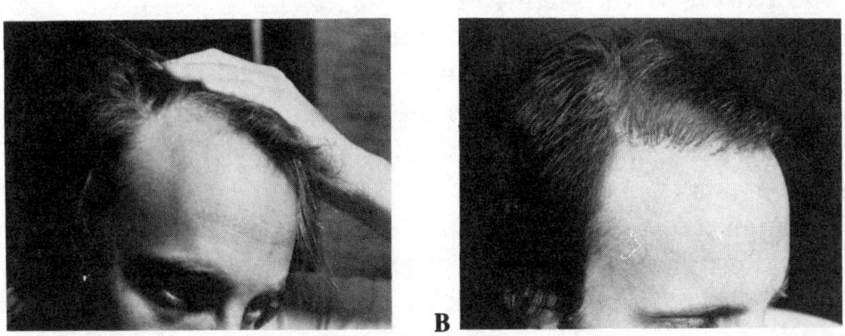

A B

Figure 6-5 A. A 28-year-old with fine, light hair demonstrating loss of hair anteriorly on the right. **B.** Good coverage after 120 hair transplants performed over a one year period. Another procedure will fill in the small gaps and give a thicker density.

standing out in a crowd. I'd like to get enough hair on top so that I could get lost among a group of people. I'd also like to meet a new patient and not get the feeling that she is making scalp contact with me instead of eye contact."

As he related his story, it was obvious that his baldness was severely restricting his personality, for he was shy and apologetic in speech. It took a great effort for him to look directly at the surgeon. It appeared that he also felt guilty over his apparent vanity, and was embarrassed to relate his problem. He was a twenty-nine-year-old male who looked ten years older. The area of baldness was quite extensive and I advised several bald-area reductions (a procedure described in the next section of this chapter). Thereafter, hair transplants would be performed to fill in the remaining bald areas. His horseshoe fringe of hair was wide and luxuriously thick.

Three bald-area reductions were so effective that only a small area at the frontal hairline remained, and this was studded with transplants over a four-month period.

These procedures dramatically changed his life. With a full head of hair (and it was thick and wavy) he appeared handsomer, younger, and more vital . . . and he began to act accordingly. He became more outgoing and now when he entered the office he bantered with the office staff, whereas in the past he had been quiet and almost morose. The conversation with my receptionist obviously went further than banter for they later became engaged and subsequently married. David got more hair and a new life—I lost a good receptionist.

There Are More Ways Than One . . .

Another surgical technique for hair redistribution consists of grafting strips of hair-bearing skin instead of small plugs. This was frequently performed to establish the frontal hairline, after which punch grafts filled the gaps behind it. Many physicians have tried it but have abandoned it because of its many disadvantages. Hair loss was high, the surgeon was unable to direct the hair into a natural pattern, and the hairline produced was very sharp in contrast to the natural soft, irregular line.

Other surgical procedures for baldness are the small-flap and delayed-flap operations. Both of these yield better density and immediate hair coverage as the circulation to the hair roots is maintained and there is no hair fallout. Also, unlike transplants, there are no changes in hair texture.

The short- or small-flap procedure is performed in the office and is used mainly to establish a new hair line. In essence, a tonguelike flap of hair-bearing skin, with its circulation based at the temple, is outlined on the right side. It is then cut out, rotated, and sutured into the frontal hairline, where bald skin has been removed to accept the flap. After extensive freeing of the donor area from the underlying tissue, it is closed and a large bandage is applied. This is replaced the next day with a smaller one. By the fourth day, all bandages are discarded and within one week, all sutures have been removed. Pain is minimal and only mild analgesics are needed.

Disadvantages are: (1) Although the flap carries its own blood supply, a slough may occur with consequent loss of a portion of the hair-bearing skin. This skin loss would require further remedial surgery with results that might not be too pleasing. (2) Touch-up procedures are also generally required at the base end of the flap to remove the bulging (dog ear) that can develop when the flap is turned on itself. (3) The scar along the frontal hair line may persist for three to six months; and (4) only one side can be done at a time since it is impossible to close both donor areas without undue tension. Thus, it is hard to camouflage the unoperated frontal hair line. Approximately six to eight weeks later, the opposite side can be restored.

The delayed-flap technique is used to cover a large bald area. Years ago, a person with this type of alopecia would be refused treatment because the wide area required many transplants and few had an adequate donor region to accommodate that large an area. This technique offers the same advantages and disadvantages as the small-flap procedure. However, this is a longer and wider flap and the blood supply must be secured. Therefore, extra steps are involved. These are accomplished as office procedures wherein the flap is outlined surgically and immediately resutured. The same procedure is performed again, one week later. Interruption of the circulation (the delay phenomenon) allows the flap to adapt to a lessened blood supply. One week after the last delay, the patient is admitted to the hospital for the definitive surgery. Under a local or general anesthetic, the bald area corresponding to the mirror image of the delay pattern is removed. Then the flap is lifted from its bed, rotated, and sewn into that defect (Figure 6-6). The donor defect is closed as in the small-flap approach and a similar head dressing is applied. The postoperative course is also much the same, but

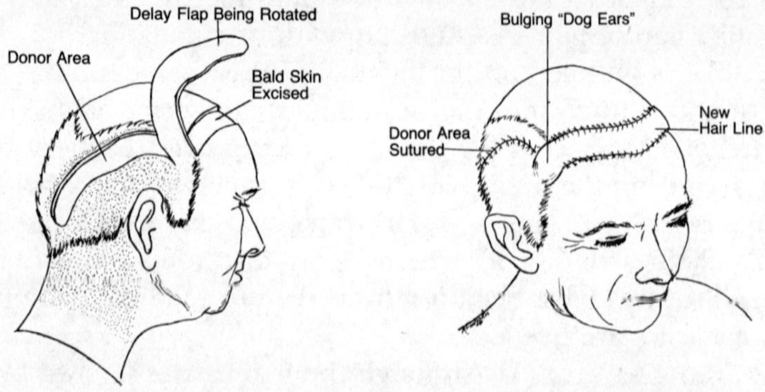

Figure 6-6 A. The delay flap is lifted from the donor area and rotated into the frontal defect. The stippled area demonstrates the amount of undermining needed in the scalp and neck to effect closure. **B.** Donor area closed and flap sewn into position. At a later date, the opposite side will be rotated into position behind this flap.

since there is more extensive surgery, more swelling and discomfort can occur. Several months later this operation can be repeated from the opposite side; it takes more than one procedure to cover the entire head.

The flap procedures definitely have their place in the treatment of baldness, but obviously are more involved and carry more serious complications. The surgical cost for the small-flap surgery is $2000 to $2500 per session and $3000 to $4000 per session for the delayed-flap operation.

The simplest way to treat extensive areas of baldness is to remove surgically as much bald area as possible. Since the skin of the scalp is flexible, the gap left by excision can be readily closed. As the bald area is reduced, there is a corresponding reduction in the number of hair transplants required for coverage. Scalp reduction is an office procedure and is now considered routine for those with large areas of baldness (Figure 6-7).

The cost of the procedure is approximately $900 to $1200. Within six weeks from the time of surgery, hair transplantation can be initiated. Most always the scalp can be operated upon again, removing yet another bald gap, which in turn further decreases the number of transplants required. In some cases, an entire bald gap can be closed after several reductions. The small scar that results from the surgery is eradicated as hair plugs are

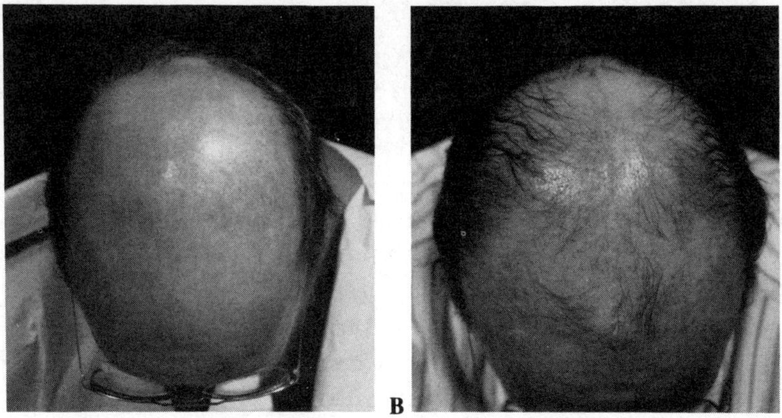

A B

Figure 6-7. A. Large area of alopecia. **B.** Baldness narrowed considerably after three scalp reductions. Will require one more reduction and hair transplantation to give adequate cover. The minimal scar will be easily covered by hair transplants.

studded into that line, completely covering it. This process not only shortens the length of time for a complete transplantation, but lessens the expense as well.

Hair In, Hair Out

While thousands of men are spending their dollars to get hair, millions of women are spending even more dollars to get rid of hair. The hair growth that occurs on the female face has many variations. Almost every young woman, upon emerging from her teens has some hair on her face. The soft down of the face is not to be considered a blemish, but part of a prized complexion. It is when the hair becomes very coarse on the upper lip and chin that it becomes a problem to women.

Sometimes It's Forever

Unwanted hair can be temporarily removed by shaving, plucking, or by depilatories. None of these methods affects hair growth. The woman who begins shaving unwanted hairs and then notices increased growth in the shaved areas may believe that her use of the razor has promoted this. Not so. The additional hairs would have emerged in any event; the common belief that shaving accelerates and increases hair growth is false.

Plucking may be harmful as it can damage tissues near the hair root; continued irritation of these tissues is instrumental in the formation of ingrown hairs and causes the possible death of hair roots. If a hair is to be plucked, the skin should be softened with a hot face towel and then the hair plucked quickly and firmly in the direction of its growth. After plucking, full regrowth is usual—eighteen weeks for scalp hair, three months for chin hair, and about two months for the eyebrows. Depilatories, like shaving, leave the face rather shiny for its natural "mat," the "peach fuzz" is removed along with the coarse hairs.

Women often ask if a face-peel will rid them of unwanted face hair. Since the hair root lies deep in the dermis, any process that would destroy it would be very destructive and cause scarring. Neither facial chemosurgery nor abrasion should cause temporary or permanent removal of hair.

The only safe way to remove hair permanently is by electrolysis. In this method the technician introduces a delicate wire into the opening of the hair follicle and applies a light current that destroys the root. Electrolysis sessions are lengthy, uncomfortable, tedious, and expensive. And if improperly applied, the current can damage the skin with resultant scarring. Also, a certain amount of hair regrowth always follows electrolysis—about 15 percent to 20 percent—as it is sometimes difficult to ascertain the follicular angle and the proper amount of current to destroy the hair root. The cost per half-hour session is about $35 to $50.

The Proper Care

Regular brushing of the hair can produce beneficial results because the procedure unknots tangles more gently than a comb and distributes the natural oils more evenly, thus adding lustre to the hair. Since the tensile strength of hair is lessened when wet, it should be brushed when it is dry to avoid breakage. In most of us, blood circulation through the scalp is adequate for all hair needs. Massage, by brushing or other means, affords a degree of pleasure and is mainly of psychological value.

More dirt collects on the hair within a twenty-four-hour period than on any other part of the body. Shampoo hair whenever it is dirty. If that is every day, then shampoo it every day. When soap, rather than a detergent shampoo is used, the application of lemon or vinegar rinses helps to remove any residual film by counteracting the alkalinity of the soap and reducing any oiliness of the scalp, thus brightening the hair. The natural action of lemon, however, can lighten hair shade over a period of time.

Hair should look like hair. It is beautiful if one allows it to be natural. It is basically a lustrous fabric and can dazzle a doorpost if treated with care. If not respected—if it is forced to do something it wasn't meant to do—it is no longer hair; it's a mess. Some of the punishment that hair is subjected to could literally curl your hair. It is bleached and dyed into unbelievable shades, sprayed and lacquered practically into stone. It is oiled, baked, waxed, and singed. It is pulled, popped, teased, and split. It is perfumed, powdered, and pampered into any one of a hundred styles with ribbons, flowers, and beads adorning it. Yet it calmly endures these tortuous practices for believe it or not, it is really quite difficult to injure; to do so takes dedicated effort.

Without a doubt, if hair did not tug sensually at our primitive emotions, no one would take heed if it grew or didn't grow; was gray, black, brown, or blonde; or whether or not it grew in parts of the body ordinarily smooth. Women have long understood that hair is a major lure in their sexual quest and have cared for it as the cosmetic treasure that it is. Only recently, however, have men come to the same understanding.

In the last two decades there has been a veritable revolution in the attitude of men to hair loss. Wigs are so accepted by women that it is possible for them to wear them merely because it is "chic." Men are not anywhere close to the point where they can be casual about wearing a hairpiece. Instead, many are taking the attitude that it is no longer necessary to be bald. Today, with the help of the cosmetic surgeon, more men are undergoing a hair-raising experience without turning a hair.

Q&A

When should I undertake hair transplantation?

There are only two reasons not to start hair transplants—when the patient is not bald enough or when he is too bald. If the hair is thinning but gives cover, hair transplants should not be done. If the area of alopecia is large, the patient may need flap procedures or scalp reduction of the bald area.

Can I return to work right after my hair transplants?

No. The head is bandaged immediately after the procedure and it is best to have a quiet time that day. The following day when the bandage is removed, one may resume nonstrenuous work.

Should I shampoo my hair every day?

Frequent shampooing reduces surface oil that may contain high levels of male hormone that could reenter the skin and adversely affect the hair follicle. Daily shampooing also rids the hair of the dirt it accumulates each day.

Should I consider hair transplantation if I have a large area of baldness?

If the bald area is extensive but you have a good horseshoe fringe of hair, the best course to follow is to remove surgically as much bald area as possible and later proceed to transplants for definitive cover-up. This is the simplest method to obtain hair coverage without going into extensive flap procedures.

What is the best method to remove unwanted hair?

For permanent removal, electrolysis. For temporary removal, shaving.

7
The Chin: Is Yours a Knockout?

Together, the nose, chin, and forehead constitute the three most important balancing masses of the face, and an intriguing intimacy exists among them. The chin is the fixed focal point to the eyes of those who look at us. It also marks the bottom line of the face and the upper terminal of the neck and throat. Thus, when the chin is too small or too large, not only is the facial architecture thrown out of balance, but the graceful line of the neck is also disrupted. A person with a small or receded chin may find life an uphill battle. Others may think that he is weak or timid and not to be entrusted with a position demanding aggressiveness. A receded chin can also exaggerate the physical prominence of the nose, as can a marked slope of the forehead. To refashion the forehead is not feasible whereas shaping the chin is. Chin redesigning to improve facial imbalance is an operation known as mentoplasty.

Common Chin Problems

The most common chin problem seen by the cosmetic surgeon is a small or receded chin (microgenia). This occurs in a child most commonly from nasal obstruction caused either by enlarged adenoids, which can prevent nasal breathing, or by blockage of the nasal airway itself (see chapter 2). The resultant mouth breathing is not the normal pattern. If continued mouth breathing occurs during development, it disrupts the opposing and balancing action of muscles that tends to promote harmonious skeletal development. When the mouth is closed, the tongue, which is a very powerful muscle, exerts upward pressure against the palate and opposes any action of the facial muscles on the palate. With the mouth open, the tongue does not push up against the palate, but lies on the floor of the mouth. This allows the action of the facial muscles to go unopposed and they compress the normal flat arch of the palate into a narrow gothic shape. As the palate becomes narrowed, it produces a receded chin as well as dental disturbances such as crowded teeth and occasionally an abnormal bite (malocclusion).

Malocclusion is the failure of the upper and lower teeth to meet appropriately when the mouth is closed. During early development, the condition can usually be corrected by orthodontic treatment. In the majority of cases, the receded chin is not associated with malocclusion or if present, it is not functionally disturbing.

Overdevelopment or protrusion of the chin (prognathism) is due to hereditary causes or disease and occurs less frequently than microgenia. These individuals quite often literally lead with their chin. People with this malformation can be erroneously accused of belligerence or of having a pugnacious attitude. They may have to defend themselves in situations that are really not of their making.

Prognathism spoils the balance between the upper two-thirds and the lower one-third of the face. It is almost always accompanied by malocclusion, with the lower teeth forward of the corresponding upper teeth. This produces problems with eating and therefore the prognathic individual has both a functional and an aesthetic problem.

Surgical Correction

A Chip Off the Old Block

The malocclusion associated with prognathism determines the amount of surgery required. Under general anesthesia, a segment of jaw is cut out on each side and the jaw is slid backward into the space thus created. This effectively alleviates the "bite" problem and corrects the protruding jaw. The operating time is several hours and the hospital stay several days.

Whenever the jaw is split, it must be wired together to ensure proper healing of the bones. The dental wires remain approximately six weeks, during which time the patient is on a liquid or semisoft diet. Convalescence is more involved than in chin augmentation since bone segments are removed and the jaws must be immobilized to allow for healing.

Chin Up

When augmentation of the chin is indicated, it can be

performed at the same time as a rhinoplasty without any added convalescence. When a large nose and a small chin are placed in the hands of the cosmetic surgeon, the combined effect of the two corrective procedures is electrifying for quite literally, a new look is carved upon the face (Figure 7-1).

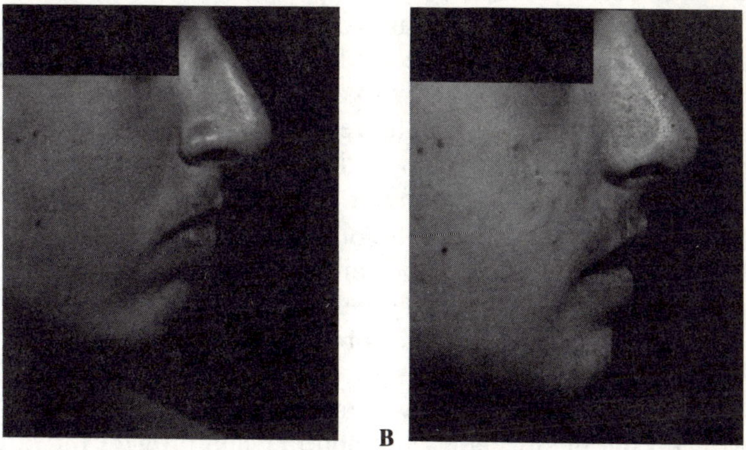

A B

Figure 7-1 A. Large nose and retruded chin. **B.** Dramatic change following rhinoplasty and chin implant—one week postoperative.

This new look does not always completely change one's life as this story illustrates. Twenty-year-old Sally was referred to me by her physician. She had been in therapy for severe depression. Along with recounting her unhappy family life, she had related to her therapist how hopelessly ugly she thought she was. "When I'm here, I seem to feel better as we talk about my situation, but when I walk outside that door, nothing has changed about my nose and chin. No matter how much we talk about it, they don't change." That her appearance was a contributing factor to her dark moods was not overlooked by her therapist, who felt that perhaps a new look might lessen some of Sally's problems.

Her first session with me showed how deep her feelings about herself were. "With no chin and a big nose, I feel like a figure in a cartoon and yet I have to face real situations. No wonder nobody will go with me. I don't know how anyone can stand to look at me. My mother tells me that the right man will love me just as I am. What a joke! How can a man love me when *I* don't even love me . . ." and with that she burst into tears.

During this interview and in several successive visits, it became apparent that she had suffered severely during her childhood. An unstable home life and the lack of affection from two immature, alcoholic parents had produced an anxious, insecure, and unloved girl. She had no social life, not even a close girl friend to whom she could confide her secrets or fantasies.

After an unsuccessful suicide attempt, she had been channeled to a psychiatrist, who was her only vocal outlet for her feelings of depression about herself and the world. Although very unhappy, she was a self-supporting social worker and was presently involved in work with the mentally retarded. This was her deliberate choice since she believed that these children would not find a person like her unappealing.

Sally was a very passive and nervous woman who was constantly fidgeting with her hands and face. Initial scrutiny revealed that she was also very homely with a large, hooked nose and a markedly receded chin. Her profile gave the visual impression of a dull, languid person, a fact quickly repudiated upon conversation with her. However, when the profile was redrawn with the bump shaded out and the chin brought forward, something else came forth. From that slumbering silhouette, emerged a dynamic look. What was drawn at the office was executed in surgery. Her convalescence was routine and she emerged far more attractive than she had ever dreamed she could be. She loved the way that she now looked and I felt that the successful cosmetic repair might alleviate some of her depression.

My hopes were not realized. Although the emotional drain about her looks was removed, it did not lessen her depression. Improving her appearance merely shifted energy expended on her features and gave additional time for her to dwell on her obsessive feelings about her parents and siblings. She had complained vocally about her appearance, but that was only the tip of the iceberg; her familial conflict was profound and the consuming issue in her life. After many months she did develop a relationship with a man that gave her some happiness, but when I last spoke with her therapist, she stated that Sally was still deeply involved in and dependent upon therapy. Sally continued to have difficulty integrating her self- and body-image, and was struggling to overcome her anxious and depressive feelings.

How It's Done

In the majority of cases, a receded chin is corrected by a

silicone implant. An ideal implant should be chemically and physically stable, flexible, shapable, inert, lightweight, nonallergenic, and virtually indestructible. At present, medical-grade silicone is the material with all these properties and the most common implant in chin augmentation.

The implant can be introduced using local analgesia through two different approaches. Either approach is acceptable, depending on the surgical factors and the patient's feelings about a small scar beneath his or her chin.

With the intraoral approach (internal), the surgeon makes a small incision in the gulley between the gums and lip. He frees the membranes and attached muscles from the bone and makes a pocket to house the implant. An implant that has been carved to the patient's needs is slipped into the pocket and the wound is closed. Although this approach eliminates an external scar, there is a greater risk of contamination from oral fluids and it is therefore not recommended for persons with poor dental hygiene.

With the external route, a horizontal incision about one inch long is made just beneath the chin in a crease found in most people. The surgeon makes a pocket large enough to accommodate the implant and after inserting it, closes the wound. Neither approach causes much bleeding. Total time for either operation is approximately thirty minutes. With either procedure, a small pressure dressing is applied for several days to immobilize the implant, to inhibit oozing, and to minimize the swelling. The implant itself inhibits postoperative oozing as it exerts pressure along the entire length of the internal wound.

Postop Care

A semisoft or liquid diet is recommended for the first few days following surgery since it is difficult to chew. Analgesics are also prescribed for the discomfort. Those who have undergone the intraoral route must observe strict oral hygiene. Mouth washes are advocated. The intraoral sutures are self-dissolving and are absorbed in several weeks. To discourage infection the surgeon prescribes antibiotics, which are discontinued after one week. Men should not shave for approximately one week to avoid disturbing the implant. Two or three weekly follow-up office visits are routine. Mucous membranes repair themselves quickly and after a few weeks, the intraoral incision will be healed. The external incision necessitates suture removal and takes longer to heal. The scar will eventually blend into the natural submental

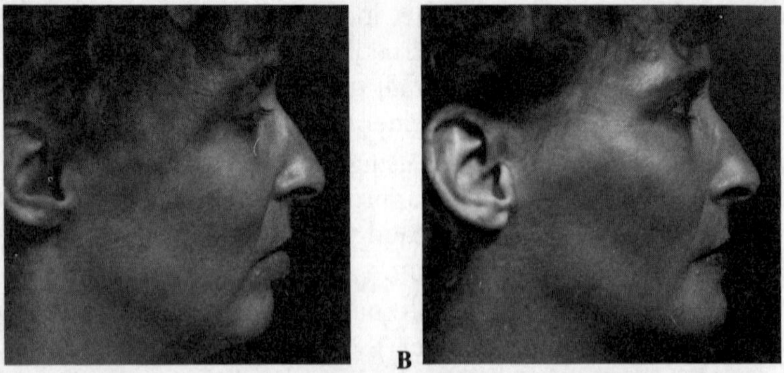

A B

Figure 7-2. A. Receded chin, moderate degree. **B.** Intraoral placement of implant gives a stronger, more attractive profile—two months postoperative.

(underchin) creases within several months. Implantation is an office procedure or, if preferred, it can be performed in a hospital on an out-patient basis. As shown by Figures 7-2 and 7-3, remarkable improvements are obtainable with a chin implant.

Complications from the surgery are infrequent. The most common is an infection which, if not controlled, will cause rejection of the implant. Even if rejection occurs and the implant must be removed, if several months have elapsed since surgery, the new chin profile will essentially retain its shape since the

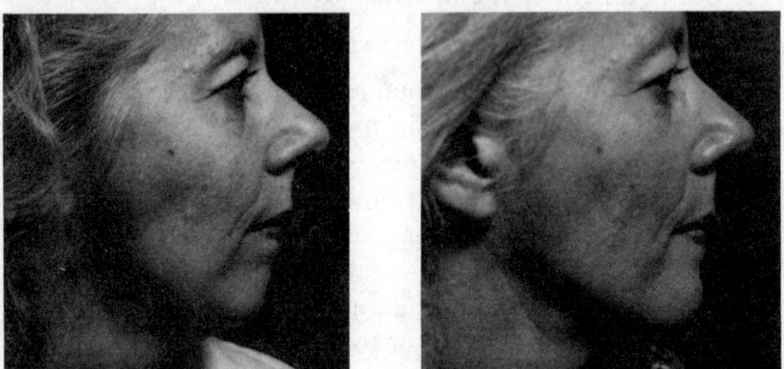

A B

Figure 7-3 A. Receded chin, severe degree. **B.** Placement of large intraoral implant creates a much prettier chin line—five months postoperative (nose has never been operated upon).

cavity tends to fill in with scar tissue, which adds volume to the chin. Also, the overlying skin and muscles, which have adapted to the presence of the implant by stretch and realignment, will not completely fall back to their original posture.

This Dent Can Leave You With a Favorable Impression

A cleft or dimple in the chin adds piquancy to the face, and frequently will soften a large chin. A natural chin dimple occurs almost exactly in the midline and takes the shape of a vertical furrow. It can be duplicated within thirty minutes as an office procedure under local analgesia. The surgeon makes a small half-inch incision just under the chin. He then passes a tiny scissors upward toward the mark made for the new dimple and frees the skin under the dimple site from the underlying muscle. Next, he introduces a small blade through this original incision line and cuts the muscle and underlying tissue all the way to bone. As the cut muscle and tissue spread apart, this creates a small space. The skin is now pressed downward and held in place by a small mold that is sewn into place. The incision is closed with several sutures; no bandaging is required. When the pressure mold is released two days later, the union between the skin and bone has created a depression. The beauty of this manufactured dimple is that no scar is visible in the furrow. Also, if the impression is too deep, it can be massaged for several minutes over the next few days; this will break down some of the adhesions that are forming and produce a more shallow dimple (Figure 7-4).

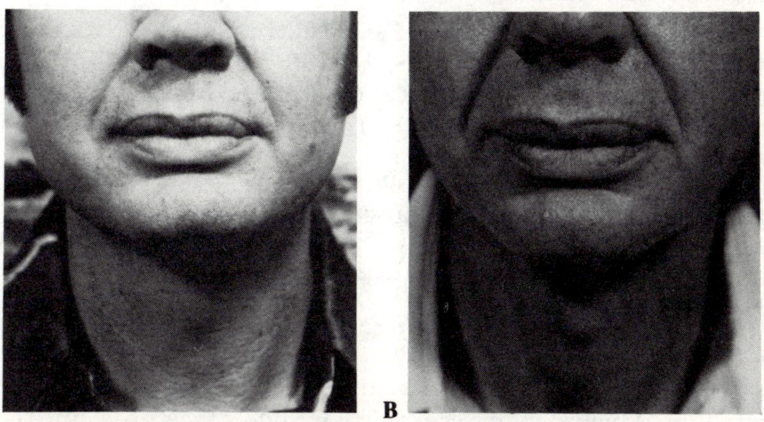

A B

Figure 7-4 A. Wide, full chin. **B.** Subtle cleft imparts a softer look to the chin.

Lips Are for Love

Second only to the eyes, the lips comprise the other most prominent feature of the face exemplifying emotion and expression. Lips are probably the first part of the body to be decorated to increase attractiveness and even in ancient times, the allure of luscious, beautiful lips were visibly recognized (Figure 7-5). Full red lips and a prominent mouth are the hallmarks of youth; recessed thin lips suggest old age. Lips are used for sexual signaling, and in races where the color contrast with the skin is lost, larger lips have evolved, as for example in black people. Lips also permit sucking, whistling, blowing, spitting, and are the

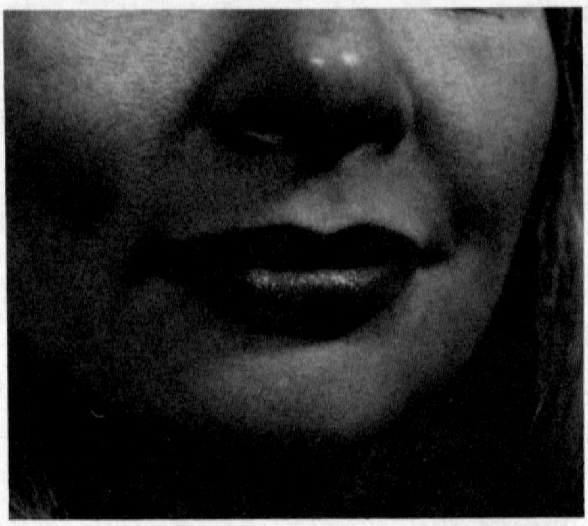

Figure 7-5 Full, luscious lips are sensual and impart a youthful look.

valve-like mechanism by which we take in food and drink. All cultures use the lips in communication and for divergent forms of sex.

Too Full or Too Thin: Surgery Can Help

Enlargement of the lips (machrocheilia) is generally confined to the red border of one or both lips. This can be decreased by removing a strip of tissue along its entire length. The wound edges are then closed with sutures. Although a moderate amount of swelling occurs following surgery, it disappears within a few weeks with little tell-tale evidence that the lips have been operated on. Machrocheilia is a thirty minute office procedure performed under local analgesia.

Thin lips can be made full and more sensuous by injections of silicone. Minute amounts of silicone fluid are introduced into either lip over several sessions. The injections are performed in the office, require no analgesic as they are virtually painless, and are well tolerated by the tissues.

Whether thin or full, the lips are central to the smile, probably the most dynamic facial expression. Smiles are all different, but ideally should show only the teeth or include only the barest portion of the gums above the teeth. When the full gums show with smiling, it produces a horsey or "gummy" look. This is usually due to a short upper lip and/or "buck" teeth protruding forward against the lips. A relatively uncomplicated, under-one-hour operation can correct this.

The surgeon removes a horizontal strip of mucous membrane extending from second molar to second molar in the gulley between the gum and upper lip. He then frees the lip flap from its underlying attachments and turns it downward to the lower portion of the incision along the gum, where he sutures it into this new position. The scar tissue seal that develops between the raw surface of the lip and the gum eliminates the overexcursion of the lip during smiling or laughing.

A plaster-of-paris splint applied over the area immobilizes the lip. This is worn for approximately one week. During this time soft foods and mouth rinses are recommended as the lip will be quite swollen and difficult to move. Pain is minimal and relieved by standard analgesics; antibiotics are given to prevent any infection. The swelling and bruising fade rapidly after one week. With this simple procedure, the lowering of the upper lip psychologically raises the patient's spirits (Figure 7-6).

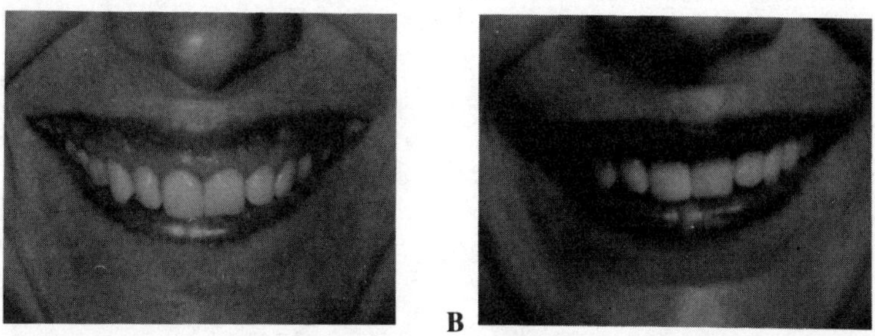

A B

Figure 7-6 A. Full denture smile bares too much gum which detracts from the smile. **B.** Full smile now shows only the teeth and the barest portion of the gum; this is a more attractive look. (Photo courtesy of Pierre Fornier, MD, Paris, France.)

What It Can Cost

Chin augmentation entails a surgical cost of $1500 to $2000. When it is performed in conjunction with a rhinoplasty, the expense can be less. Sliding a prognathic jaw back is a more complex procedure, and the fee is on the order of $3000 to $3500. The charge for reducing enlarged lips ranges from $750 to $1000, and augmenting thin lips with the use of silicone fluid costs approximately $50 per injection. $1500 is the usual surgical fee for lowering the upper lip. Prognathic surgery is classified as a medical problem and is covered by insurance; the rest are not.

Many individuals are not aware of a receded chin as they do not see themselves in profile. However, almost all individuals who know they have this defect are pleased with the improvement effected by a chin implant. Not many operations can claim such marvelous statistics. The reasons for the success of mentoplasty, besides the pleasing permanent change in the silhouette, can be found in its ease and speed of execution, lack of complications, and minimal scars. Many people have ignored the chin in the belief that its solid and rigid structure exempted it from surgery, or that chin augmentation was a jaw-breaker. Quite frankly, cosmetic operations on the chin and lips are generally simple, swift, and successful. As knowledge of this becomes more widespread, more and more people are visiting the cosmetic surgeon and taking a lick on the chin.

Q&A

Can my chin be corrected at the same time as my nose?

Yes. You can recuperate from both procedures at the same time and the convalescence is not basically prolonged by doing both.

Will my chin feel different with the implant in it?

No. The implant when buried beneath the skin is imperceptible from the patient's tissues and is indistinguishable by feel and sight.

What are the chances that the implant will be rejected?

There is always that risk. However, silicone implants are quite inert and evoke little reaction when placed within the body. Therefore, the risk of rejection is marginal.

Should I have a dimple put in my chin?

If your chin is somewhat large and protruding, creating a dimple in the skin overlying that protrusion blunts the projection of the bony chin and produces a softer look. This is much simpler than removing the projecting bone and often creates the same effect.

Will a blow to my chin crack or break the implant?

No. Implants are a thick resin substance usually of solid silicone and are quite malleable. Your bony jaw can break from a hard blow but the implant will not.

8
The Ears—Outstanding Is Not Better

The external ear (the auricle), our second most important sense organ, functions as a sound-directing device, channeling vibrations toward the eardrum, which transmits them to the hearing nerve. Because the need for this function has been declining over the centuries, the ear has become smaller and smaller. Given time, its role may be solely as a support for glasses or as a convenient hook for ornaments. Although mute and expressionless, this convoluted masterpiece plays an important part in the ensemble of a beautiful woman.

Anatomy—It's Got Some Nice Curves

The ear is comprised of cartilage, fat, and skin. In front, no fatty layer exists, and the skin hugs the cartilaginous framework tightly. On the back surface, the skin is more flexible due to a layer of fat beneath it. Several poorly developed muscles are attached to the front and back surfaces. Many animals (for example, horses, dogs, and cats) possess well-developed auricular muscles and can direct the ears toward the source of sound; however, these muscles are, for the most part, vestigial in humans, reminders of an early, more primitive era. In some people, however, these muscles are relatively well developed, and can be contracted and relaxed causing their ears to wiggle.

The average length of an adult ear is about twice its width, being 3.5 centimeters across and 6.5 centimeters from top to lobe (a dimension that tends to lengthen with age due to the effects of gravity). In the same individual, the ears may differ in size (right being larger than left) and may differ in shape as well as detail. Men have larger ears than women.

The location of the ear renders it susceptible to a variety of insults. Being exposed to the heat and cold without an adequate layer of fat, the ear is readily subject to frostbite and sunburn. A blow may cause bleeding between the cartilage and skin. Because the bloody fluid is not readily absorbed, it thickens and clots and, in doing so, obliterates the normal detail of the ear. With repeated injury, thickened scar tissue can produce a deformity known as "cauliflower ear." Since there is minimal expansile tissue on the front of the ear, severe pain can arise from minor infections on that surface. A pimple within the ear canal has so little space to expand that as the inflammation progresses, it tortuously stretches the sensory nerves, producing excruciating pain.

The above notwithstanding, the ear's thin skin and rich blood supply render it a perfect tissue reservoir for skin grafts. The texture and color of the ear skin closely resemble and match those of the face. The back of the ear (where the graft is taken) is easily repaired, leaving a concealed scar, and the thinness of the graft allows it to be nourished easily at its new site.

The lobe of the ear is often pierced by the layman with little regard for aseptic technique. An infection can occur, causing pain and distortion in the lobe. Heavy earrings and the pull they exert can split the lobe. This can be repaired by cutting away the cleft edges and suturing the raw margins (Figure 8-1). The lobes should always be pierced using aseptic technique and the opening maintained with gold or silver studs. These must not be changed for approximately two weeks to allow complete healing of the channel. During this interval, the studs and the pierced sites

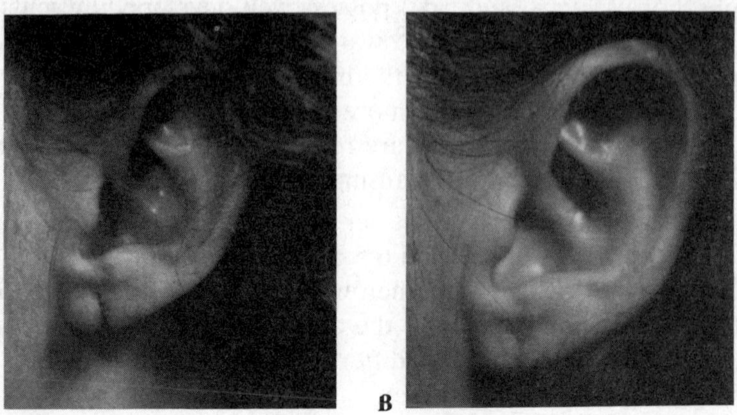

A B

Figure 8-1. A. A cleft in the earlobe from earring pull through. **B.** One month postoperative.

should be cleansed with alcohol daily, followed by application of an antibiotic ointment. After two weeks, they may be removed and any other light earring inserted. Despite the most aseptic precautions, a keloid (described in chapter 5) may develop in a susceptible individual, usually a black person. They are best treated by excision, followed by immediate doses of irradiation.

A protruding or "lop ear" is the most common ear deformity and is congenital in nature. Ear development begins at the fifth prenatal week with most malformations occurring in the third period of embryonic life. At birth, the organ is completely formed and by age three has reached three quarters of its adult size. The ear thus appears out of proportion with the head; aesthetic balance occurs with growth of the head.

Ideally, the ears should set within the middle third of the face, between the eyebrow and the base of the nose, with their long axes parallel to the nasal bridge. More important, the angle at which the ear protrudes from the side of the head (cephalo-auricular angle) should not exceed 30 degrees. If it does, the ear appears limp, stands out, and becomes lop, or protruding. Protruding ears are cosmetically disfiguring. If they are large, but set close to the head (as were Clark Gable's) they are not obtrusive. When protruding, they limit a woman's hairstyle and in men, they can impart a dull and stupid appearance to the face.

Protruding ears can also be the cause of a personality disorder and lead to unpleasant consequences, as illustrated by this case history: Phil was an inmate of a minimum security prison in California. This was his second time around—first, in his late teens for car theft and now in his mid-twenties for grand larceny and embezzlement.

In a fight with a fellow prisoner Phil had sustained a severely fractured nose. He was referred to the ear, nose, and throat clinic for evaluation of that injury.

The first thing that you noticed about Phil was his protruding ears. The second thing you noticed was the way he put his cap on, low down around his ears, snuggling them to his head, with an immediate improvement in his looks.

While being examined, he asked if his ears could be fixed. This was the first opportunity he had ever had to question someone who performed cosmetic surgery and although he could hardly breathe through his nose, he was more interested in the details of otoplasty.

He told me that because of his ears he had suffered, as a kid, from daily humiliation as the butt of endless corny jokes. His lop ears had also been the cause of many a fistfight with the other kids. He had always worn his hair long in an effort to hide them, but he could no longer do that while serving time. As he grew older, he began to initiate fights to show that he was someone to be reckoned with, and he soon became the neighborhood tough. Because of his scrappy reputation, he later became an enforcer for a shylock. This led to other underworld activities and the con game. Eventually he paid the price.

Both his ears and nose were operated upon. There was minimal change with his nose as the preponderance of work involved the inside to improve his breathing. The battening down of his ears was an elegant stroke. For the first time, he felt comfortable with a close haircut. This now gave him a cleaner, neater appearance and his rugged, virile looks were no longer marred by his comical ears.

I made many visits to this penal complex to help in the rehabilitation of the inmates and saw Phil quite often. From a discussion with the other personnel, I found out that he had become a better behaved prisoner, kinder and less pugnacious. This was noted by everyone. Whether it was due to his fear that an injury would undo all that had been done or just a real change in his personality is not known. At this writing Phil is still in prison and I don't know which way he will go when he is released. There is one thing I do know and that is how he felt when I unbandaged his ears and nose and he first looked at himself. He smiled, turned to me, and said: "Doc, you've made a friend for life."

Bend Me Your Ear

Many parents try to rectify protruding ears in their youngsters by the application of compression bandages, headbands, or adhesive strips. These methods are doomed to failure as cartilage is practically a perfect spring, and can be bent for long periods of time without permanent change. Once the bending force is removed, the cartilage will return to its original position. In the same vein, sleeping on the curled ear for great lengths of time cannot deform it. The temper of the cartilage *must* be altered to change the shape or angulation of the ear and this can only be done by an operation known as otoplasty.

Otoplasty can reduce the size of the ear and change its shape, design, or angle from the head. The toughness and resiliency of the cartilage lend themselves well to surgery and when operated upon, the tissue heals readily. Once the spring is broken, its elasticity permits a wide range of reshaping and just about any type of ear deformity can be refashioned with considerable improvement.

Although the world of the child is a very cruel one, it is best to delay surgery until the ears reach their full growth (about age seven). Because men's hairstyles are generally shorter than women's, otoplasty is performed more frequently on males. Long hairstyles in children and long hair and thick sideburns in men can often camouflage prominent ears. As hairstyles become shorter again, otoplasties will tend to increase.

This Broken Spring Will Make It Better

Many different procedures to correct protruding ears are described in the surgical journals, but all contain minor variations on the same theme. They are all fundamentally based upon (1) breaking the cartilage spring and bending it backwards to a position closer to the head and (2) in doing so, making sure that the new ear position is not plastered against the head. That way, when kids are reminded to wash behind their ears, they won't have an excuse not to.

In young children with very pliable cartilage, the spring can be weakened by serrating it through a small skin incision. The ear is then bent backwards and held in place by several retaining sutures which are removed in one week. This method obviates the need for extensive surgery or skin excisions. In older individuals, where the cartilage is stiffer and thicker, ears are corrected in this manner: (1) a crescent strip of skin is cut away from the back part of the ear; (2) several strategically placed cuts in the cartilage break the spring; (3) the limp cartilage now curls and lays back against the head at a more normal angle; (4) this curl is reinforced by several internal sutures; (5) the skin incision on the back of the ear is closed with fine suture; and (6) the new ear position is also reinforced by several external sutures, which further stabilize the newly curled cartilage. The head is turned and the opposite side operated upon.

On occasion, oversized, elongated, or unattractive earlobes must also be corrected. A surgeon quite often redesigns lobes, particularly attached ones, so that they will hide the face-lift incision line around the lobe. A lobe that is attached to the skin of the jaw is a recessive trait in Homo Sapiens, and occurs more frequently in females by a two-to-one ratio.

Shaving or trimming the hair is not necessary before surgery for a Vaseline® coat is applied to the area and this easily holds the hair away from the operative field. Children are given a general anesthetic, whereas teenagers or adults easily tolerate the procedure under a local analgesic. Under a general, it is a hospital stay of one-half day, and with a local the surgery can be performed in the office or hospital, whichever is preferred. At the completion of the surgery, which takes approximately one-and-one-half hours, a large, light dressing is applied to the ears and a snug, compression bandage is wrapped around that to ensure the new position of the ears.

This large, bulky dressing is worn for approximately four days. Upon removal, the external retention sutures, if any, are removed and a smaller, less bulky bandage is applied. This stays on for three more days, when it is discarded for good; thereafter,

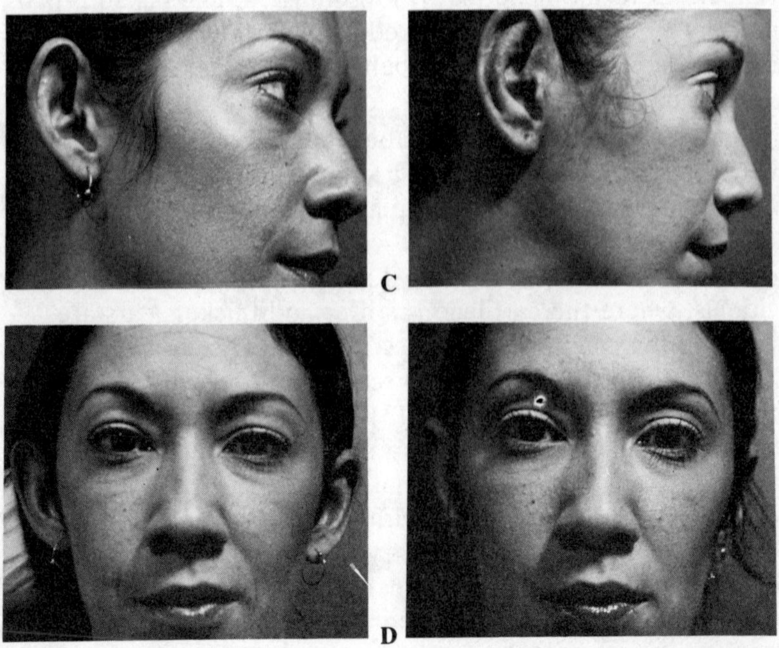

A C B D

Figure 8-2 A, B. "Lop" ears flaring away from head. **C.** Note the pleasing curve of the inner fold of the ear—six days postoperative (sutures still in place at back of the ear). **D.** Seven months postoperative.

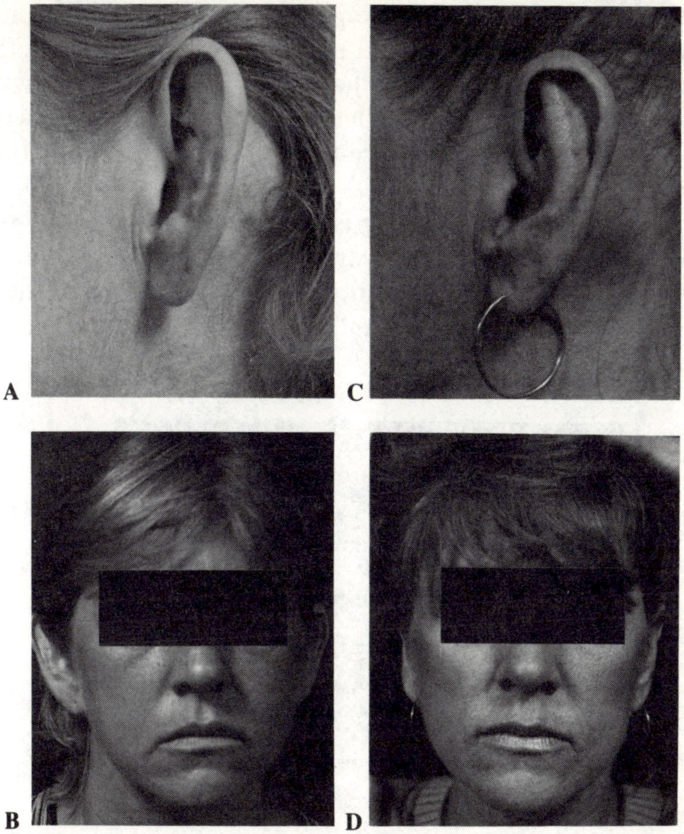

Figure 8-3 A, B. Protruding ears caused by the absence of the inner fold of the ear (antihelix). **C, D.** Laying the ear back creates this fold and produces a neater look—five months postoperative.

only a small headband is worn during sleep to prevent the ear from curling on itself in its new position. The skin sutures are removed at this time. In small children, absorbable skin sutures are used. This circumvents the unpleasant task of removing them from a possibly moving target. Only several more visits to the surgeon's office are required to follow the progress of the healing.

Postoperative pain is minimal and standard analgesics easily relieve any discomfort. An infection is rare, but always a possibility. If it were to occur, the results could be disastrous; therefore, antibiotics are prescribed.

Following the surgery, the ears will have a violaceous color for about one month from blood congestion, and some swelling for a few weeks. Because of the interference with the blood flow between the skin and cartilage, the patient should avoid extremes of heat or cold. The patient should not sunbathe or go skiing for one month, but may shampoo the hair within two weeks. Any injury to the ear during the immediate postoperative period will probably prolong the convalescence and possibly interfere with the expected result.

Occasionally the cartilage spring is not broken thoroughly and the ear, after a period of time, reverts to its previous exaggerated position. In these cases, the operation can be repeated and the cartilage earmarked for further remodeling.

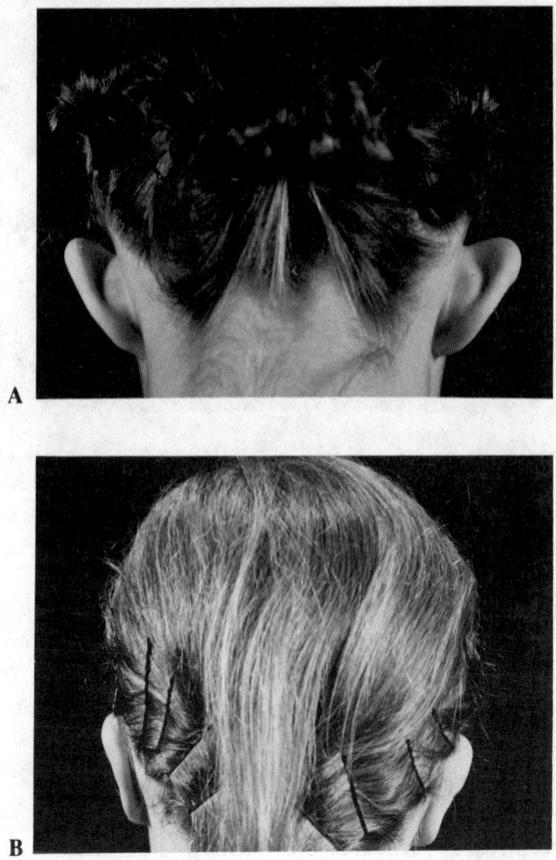

Figure 8-4 **A.** From behind note how ears flare away from the head. **B.** Postoperatively the flare disappears and the ears now hug the scalp—two years after surgery.

The most serious complications are: (1) an infection of the cartilage that could result in distortion of the ear; therefore, as stated, antibiotics are routinely prescribed; (2) a hematoma (blood accumulation beneath the skin) which, if untreated, could also misshape the ear. Treatment consists of prompt drainage of the clotted blood and the application of firm pressure dressings within the convolutions to prevent formation of scar tissue. In the main, otoplasty is an operation usually free of complications. Figures 8-2, 8-3, and 8-4 show three examples of the surgery.

Abnormally large ears (macrotia) can be reduced by removing a triangular or crescent-shaped wedge of skin and cartilage from the entire thickness of the ear. Length or width (or both) can be decreased by excisions within the ear's convolutions, thus leaving a fine to minimal scar. In cases of microtia (small or absent ear), no frame is usually available for designing the contours and depressions intrinsic to a natural ear. In these cases, many and usually complex surgeries are required. The cosmetic results are not always satisfying.

Let's Hear It for the Ears. Surgical fees for otoplasty range between $1500 and $2000. Extreme pathologies such as macrotia or microtia may entail greater expense and hospital stay; but the surgical fee, together with the cost of hospitalization, is defrayed by insurance, whereas in the case of a standard otoplasty, they usually are not.

Summary

If a deformity such as a protruding ear is not corrected in childhood or early adolescence, it is usually never corrected. By some mental gymnastics, the affected person adjusts to his deformity and to the reactions it elicits among others. Whether or not the adjustment itself provokes personality damage could be a separate topic for discussion. For unlike most other disfigurements, protruding ears generally evoke laughter, not sympathy. Continued ridicule could promote abnormal psychological development such as feelings of inadequacy and insecurity, especially in a child or vulnerable teenager. Otoplasty is a simple and expedient method of correcting the cosmetic and social nuisance known as "lop ears." The procedure is unrivaled for restoring a child's self-composure and poise for with a stroke of the scalpel, the operation can turn a clown into a ringleader.

Q&A

Can I change the angle (shape) of my child's ears by having him wear a compression bandage for a certain length of time?

No. One could wrap a bandage around the head and compress the ears inward for years and they would still flare out after an interval of time following the bandage removal. Because the ear cartilage is so rigid and so perfect a spring, its temper must be broken before the ear will lie flat and close to the head.

How soon can I shampoo my hair after surgery?

Because some type of bandaging must be worn around the ears to help maintain its new position, shampooing should be delayed for more than a week. Needless to say, you should take great care not to disturb the ear when shampooing your hair. You should continue to be extremely careful for six weeks following surgery.

Is there much pain following an otoplasty?

Since there is practically no muscle pull involving any of the features, the pain is minimal with an otoplasty, as with most facial procedures.

My ears are close to my head, but they are very large. Can their size be reduced?

Yes. In these cases, a through-and-through section of skin-cartilage-skin must be removed from each ear. This will leave an external scar that should be quite faint, but nevertheless there will be a scar that may be visible.

My ears are okay, but I have very large, hanging earlobes. Can they be fixed?

Yes. By removing a through-and-through crescent of skin-fat-skin, the lobe can be made smaller and shorter. This scar blends in very well and is rarely visible.

9
The Torso—It Can Be a Letdown

Although we are preoccupied with the head and neck since they are so obvious, body sculpting is becoming increasingly fashionable as current clothing styles lend themselves to more exposure and require less imagination. The cosmetic surgeon can remodel the breasts, flatten the belly, trim the hips, raise the buttocks, and lighten and tighten the skin of the hands and arms. In a figurative sense, once in the "body shop," he can take a woman with the chassis of a dump truck and "hammer" her into a Ferrari.

The Bosom—Its Rise and Fall

The breasts form the dominant and focal points of the female figure and they stand out as the most common torso structure operated upon. They are organs of limited physiological importance, but have gained a social significance of monumental proportions. Many young women look upon their breasts as the prime indicator and foremost symbol of their sexual desirability.

We are born either male or female; however, we become masculine or feminine through the pressures of our culture. Teenage girls first identify their femininity with the appearance of their breasts. If abnormal in size or shape, they may spawn feelings of embarrassment over their body-image and sexual inadequacy, with devastating psychologic consequences.

For the flat-chested woman, the psychological need for a fuller bust-line can develop into an obsession. The advertising media have glorified the breasts to the point where the average female may suffer an inferiority complex if she is less endowed than the currently reigning model or actress. And dress designers are continually engrossed with bosom emphasis for it is the essential element in attractiveness, whether in bathing suits or fashionable dresses.

Through the years, women have tried to enlarge their breasts by investing in creams, hormones, pills, massages, vitamins, vibrating and suction machines, exercise devices and, when these have ultimately failed, the padded bra. Actually, the only long-lasting way to achieve any increase in the breast size is by an operation known as augmentation mammaplasty.

Take Two, They're Small

Currently, all augmentation surgery is performed with implants of silicone gel, saline, or a combination of both. They closely simulate the consistency of the breast and are available in various sizes. Their flexibility allows them to be folded for insertion through a rather small incision and their inertness minimizes the foreign-body reaction.

One or both breasts can be augmented. Minor variations in breast size and contour are common, but in some instances, a gross asymmetry may be present. The underdevelopment of one breast can occur through inadequate hormonal stimulation or because its growth has been restricted by a tumor or infection; in many cases, the cause of developmental asymmetry is never known. If both breasts are small but asymmetrical, a larger implant is placed in the smaller of the two to gain equality of size and contour. If one breast is adequate, only the smaller one receives an implant.

The Surgical Procedure requires approximately one to one-and-a-half hours, and is performed under local or general anesthesia. After the patient is prepped and draped, the surgeon marks the mid-portion crease between the breast and abdomen and makes a two-inch incision just below and parallel to that mark. When the breast is enlarged by the implant, this incision will be pulled upward into the immediate fold beneath the breast where it will camouflage the scar. The dissection is carried beneath the breast to the tissue overlying the chest muscles, creating a pocket just large enough to accommodate the implant. The implant is introduced and sandwiched between the mammary tissue and the chest wall. Proper location of the implant is accomplished by manual adjustment; it need not be surgically secured as it cannot shift in the snug recess.

In many cases, the areola (the pigmented area surrounding the nipple) can be incised in a semilunar fashion and the implant inserted through this avenue (the circum-areolar approach). The implant size, in some cases, excludes this route for large silicone gel implants, as these cannot be slipped through this site without ripping the incision area. The areolar approach is ideal, however, for the saline inflatable bag prosthesis. The deflated bag can be wedged through a small incision and filled with saline to the desired volume. The major drawback of this implant is that in some cases, it loses some of its volume and becomes smaller with time. Apparently by osmosis, the saline passes through the semipermeable membrane that encloses the fluid, for when the bag is removed and inspected, no tear or rent can be found. This semiareolar approach leaves a scar that is barely visible; however, it is not uncommon for a patient to have a temporary loss of nipple sensation for several weeks.

After wound closure, the breasts are either wrapped with a circumferential bandage or placed immediately into a bra—at the discretion of the surgeon. The patient is at bed rest, but may walk on the day of surgery. If the surgery takes place in the office, she may return home after several hours in the recovery room. The triad of pills prescribed upon discharge includes pain, sleep, and antibiotic medication.

If the breasts are bandaged, the dressing is removed the next day and replaced with a loose-fitting bra, which, although changed from time to time, is worn awake and asleep for two weeks. Suture removal begins in one week and by the tenth day all the stitches are removed. The patient may bathe the day following surgery and after one week, she may temporarily remove the brassiere to shower and shampoo. Lifting her hands above her head may produce some tenderness, but will not cause any harm. Water is permitted on the breasts, but they should not be vigorously washed. Strenuous activity is inadvisable for six weeks, although the patient's convalescent period will be only ten to fourteen days. For several weeks following surgery, sexual activity should only be engaged in with premeditated caution as excitable breast manipulation can be painful and the suture line could be disrupted.

Complications Are Rare; although rejection of the implant is the most feared outcome, its occurrence is rare. Bleeding, infection, and severe pain are uncommon. The most frequent and least understood complication is the thick scar, or capsule, that forms internally around the implant.

When a foreign substance is inserted anywhere into the body, the immune system triggers a response to this intrusion and forms a protective, fibrous wall around the object. This is precisely what occurs in breast implantation.* For most patients, this is not troublesome. However, some experience an exaggerated foreign-body reaction which produces an excessive and thick fibrous capsule around the implant. Why it occurs in some and not others, and why it may develop after several years are both unanswered questions as of this writing. As this scar capsule contracts, the breast will feel firmer than previously. The contraction can also distort the contour of the breast and, in some patients, cause pain.

Only if this capsule is large enough so that the implant is freely movable within will the implant feel soft. Therefore, the patient is instructed to move her breasts manually up and down and side to side from the first postoperative day on (Figure 9-1). This exercise is performed several times a day over several months. Despite these manipulations, some patients still develop a thick capsule.

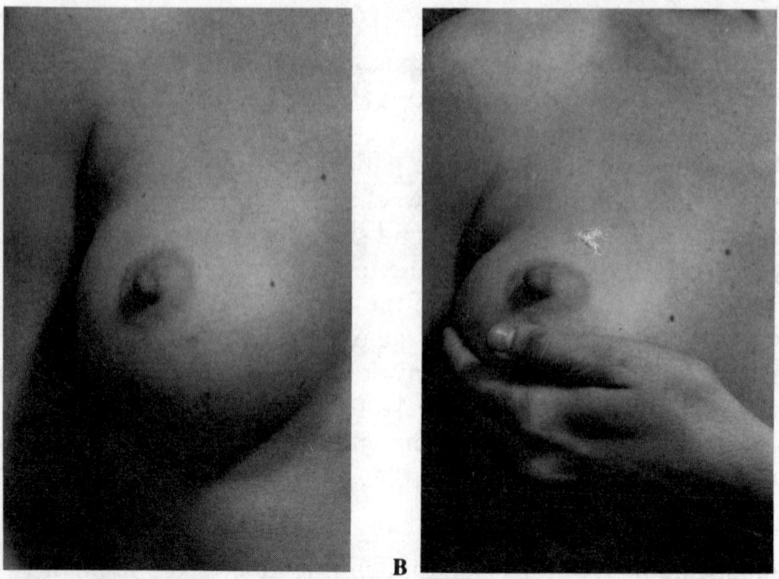

A B

Figure 9-1 A. Three times a day for several months the breasts are lifted upward and allowed to fall back into their natural position. This is performed twenty times in the 10 o'clock, 12 o'clock, and 2 o'clock positions. **B.** The breast is raised into the 12 o'clock position.

Implants in the cheek, nose, and chin also form capsules, but these are normally firm areas and cause no cosmetic disturbance.

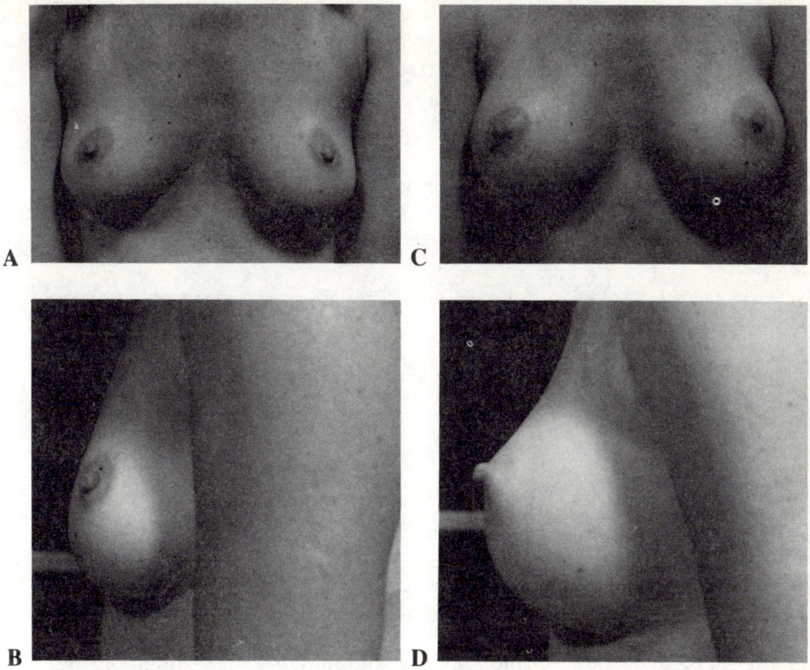

Figure 9-2 A, B. Moderate sag and minimal forward thrust. **C, D.** Three months following silicone gel implantation via inframammary approach.

Occasionally, the surgeon can break the capsule apart by manual compression. However, this maneuver could possibly rupture the implant, which would necessitate an emergency surgical intervention and implant removal. If the capsule cannot be ruptured with firm, steady pressure, it is unwise to continue with massive compression. The patient should be reoperated upon, the capsule surgically released, and a new implant inserted. Since the mechanism causing the fibrous capsule is unknown, there is no guarantee that another will not form.

Antibiotics are routinely given, but if an infection occurs that cannot be controlled, the chance of implant rejection becomes a reality. Under local analgesia, the implant is removed and the tissues are allowed to heal. Several months later, implantation can be retried.

Many women ask if breast implants cause cancer. Mammary implants can neither cause cancer, prevent cancer, nor cure cancer. Nor will they hinder the clinical detection of a tumor that

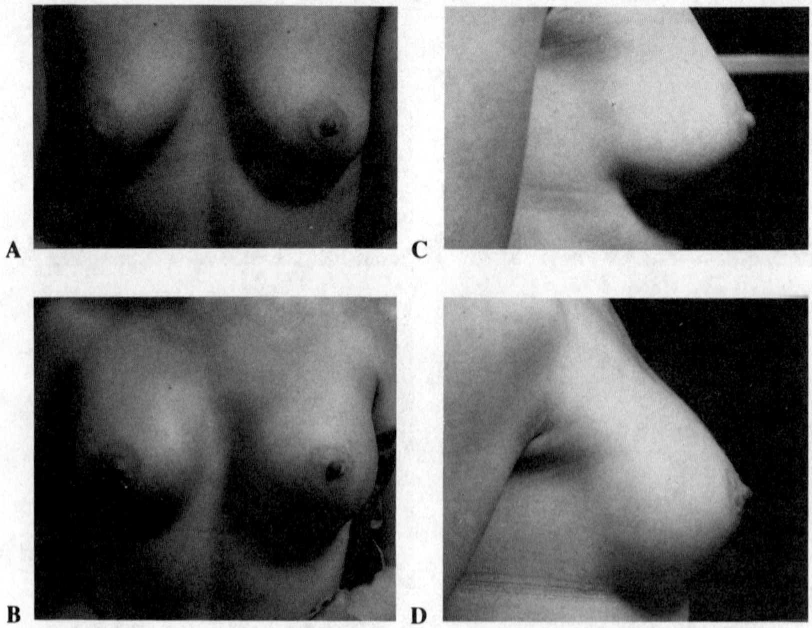

Figure 9-3 A, B. Beautifully formed breasts with minimal sag. Patient desired more cleavage and forward projection. **C, D.** Silicone gel implanted via inframammary approach—six months postoperative.

might arise after the operation as the implant is placed in a pocket behind the mammary gland; a tumor can be discovered by palpation or X-ray. Nor will the implant affect breast feeding as the surgery does not interfere with the lactating glands.

How long will an implant last? Based on laboratory studies, it should last for a lifetime. As of this time, no one has been implanted for a full life span and it is impossible to give a definite answer. Examples of breast augmentation are shown in Figures 9-2 and 9-3.

How it can change one's life is exemplified by this case history: Jeannie was a forty-five-year-old mother of three who requested breast augmentation. She related the following story: "When I was younger I had a terrific figure and beautiful breasts. With the intervening years and especially after the children, my breasts became smaller and my waist larger. That really bothered me, but it bothered my husband even more. After my last baby, he became thoroughly disenchanted and lost all interest in me sexually. On many occasions, my breasts became a focal point of bedroom argument. He would repeatedly make slurring remarks about their size. That didn't help me feel feminine or loved, and I became ashamed to show or allow them to be touched. Our marriage slowly deteriorated but we stuck it out for appearances and for the kids. After fifteen years of marriage we separated and finally divorced.

"Although that man made me feel more owned than wanted, I want to get into a serious relationship again. You can't imagine how depressing it is to be single, alone, and on the distant side of forty. But it's very difficult and emotionally disturbing for me to get sexually involved with anyone because of the inadequacy I feel about my breasts. That's why I'm here. This is the first time that I've had enough courage to do something about making them more attractive."

Examination revealed that she had lost considerable breast tissue following her pregnancies. The breasts were small, almost flat, but fortunately had minimal sag. The nipple-areolar complex was large. Her problem was amenable to breast augmentation for which a circum-areolar approach could be used. After detailed discussion regarding the merits and complications of the procedure, she was scheduled. The augmentation was performed under a general anesthetic and using a silicone prosthesis. When the bandages were removed the next day, she looked down onto an overflowing, natural-looking bosom. She discarded her padded bra. With each successive office visit, the surgeon could sense her growing self-confidence. She appeared less anxious and more at peace with herself. For her, a large measure of femininity and self-esteem had been restored. That was enough to help her develop into a stronger person and a more independent woman. The files do not record what happened to her; however, it was evident to the surgeon that with or without a relationship with a man, there would be stability in her future.

The Large, Sagging Breast

A more severe pathology is the large, pendulous, sagging breast. This not only causes emotional and social heartache because of the bust's aesthetic appearance, but leads to physical problems as well. These individuals suffer from backaches and posture defects together with deep grooves and ulcerations as the bra straps cut into their shoulders. Owing to the sensitivity of mammary tissue to hormonal stimulation, breasts can increase rapidly at puberty and become larger and sag with maturation.

This is known as "virginal hypertrophy" and the excess volume is entirely made up of glandular tissue. In post menopausal hypertrophy, the huge breast is soft and fatty with most of the glandular tissue having regressed. In postpartum breasts, the additional fat that occurs with weight gain and the increase in glandular elements during pregnancy heighten the stress on the suspensory ligaments of the breast, causing them to stretch and break down. Gravity does the rest. Correction of pendulous breasts is known as a deaugmentation mammoplasty, or mastopexy.

The Breasts Are Reduced in Size by removing excess tissue, which allows firming and elevation of the breasts. The nipple is also relocated to a higher position. Breast volume is reduced and its forward projection increased. This operation, however, involves extensive incisions that heal into an anchor-shaped scar. It circles the areola, runs vertically downward to the fold of the breast, and spreads out into a horizontal line within that fold (Figure 9-4). The procedure takes approximately three hours and

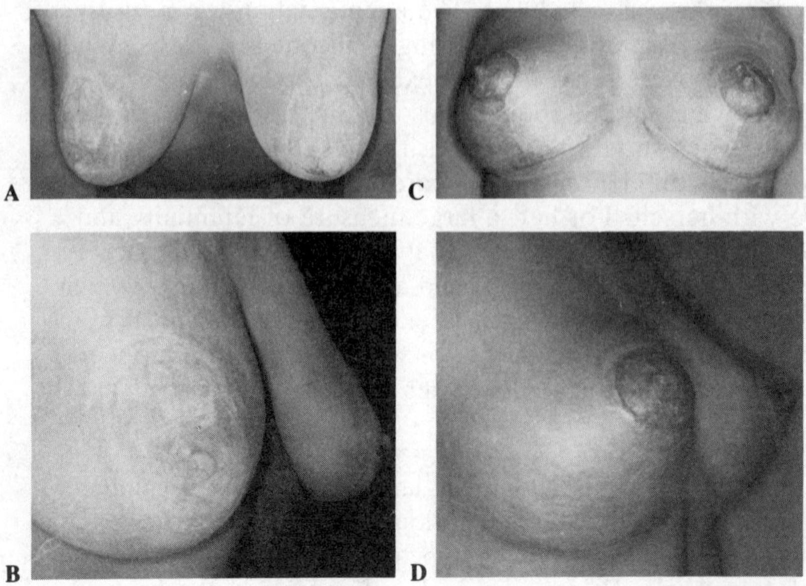

Figure 9-4 A, B. Large, pendulous breasts. **C, D.** After a mastopexy, note how much more conical and thrusting the breasts are. Also notice how much smaller the areolae are. The scars are usually more obvious due to their placement—fourteen months postoperative.

is performed under a general anesthetic; the operation may therefore be rendered inadvisable by the patient's state of health, that is, if she has heart or pulmonary disease, or other serious physiological problems.

Following the operation, the surgeon inserts drains to remove any serum that might accumulate and then applies compression bandages. The drains are removed in forty-eight hours, at which time the patient is discharged from the hospital. After two weeks, all sutures are out and the patient is instructed to wear a snug bra both when awake and asleep for one month. Antibiotics are prescribed and since more dissection has been carried out, stronger analgesics than for augmentation are needed. The convalescence is also slightly longer than for augmentation.

Although the scars are difficult to hide, most patients are extremely grateful to have the size of their breasts reduced. They not only look better, but they are no longer rigidly restricted in the choice and fashion of their clothes.

The Most Common Complication is a breakdown of the incision line which, if it occurs, results in a larger scar. The most serious complication is the loss of the nipple. If this were to occur, a portion of the vaginal labia minora would be grafted onto the nipple site. This tissue strongly resembles the nipple and aesthetically is acceptable; however, it lacks erector muscle, and will not react to stimulation.

Hey, Look Me Over

Figure trimming, or body-sculpting, below the breast comes into play because of gravity and an increase of body fat. Fat is an integral part of our bodies. Basically, there are three kinds: one kind fills in gaps between our organs and is the padding contour of the body; another is the normal reserve of fuel fat which is an energy reservoir with a high conversion ratio. These reserves, which are localized all over the body, build up when we ingest excess calories. When the nutritional income from the intestinal tract is insufficient to meet the demands of activity, these reservoirs are called upon to provide energy, with a reduction of the fat and subsequent weight loss. A third type, which is an abnormal potential reserve of fuel not easily convertible is the major cause of the pathology touted as cellulite.

Through the ages, until recently, it was the plump rather than the lean who served as models of beauty. Even now, many peoples of the Third World equate corpulence with beauty. Today, however, thinness in the American female bespeaks sensuality, whereas plumpness is associated with motherhood. This concept is as erroneous as is the tenet that big-breasted women are possessed of inordinate sexuality. However, the thin, chic woman does create more impact for she commands presence without mass and because the general view nowadays is that obesity is unaesthetic. The overweight person often appears older and less attractive. Also, the prejudice against fat people in our society is appalling and almost impossible to eradicate. Thus, the girl who overeats and becomes fat soon discovers that there is a type of heartburn other than gastronomic. She soon discovers that fat is what wallflowers are made of.

This Could Be the Start of Something Big

Of the various afflictions of the human body, obesity is the most prevalent and widespread in this country. The United States is not only the land of comfortable plenty, but also a nation of altogether too much, for one out of every three Americans overeats and is fatter than he or she should be. Some ravenous eaters do not even allow themselves to savor food on the palate—it is just short-circuited straight to their bellies. Despite the beliefs of many, this nutritional disorder is rarely glandular unless, of course, you want to consider your mouth a gland.

Millions suffer from a host of diseases directly attributable to obesity. Two such are high blood cholesterol and high blood pressure. The best way to decrease blood cholesterol in the body is to lose weight. Losing weight also lowers the blood pressure. The lower the blood pressure, the better the chances of living for *blood pressure is the single most important determinant in predicting longevity.*

Yet there are possibly more people living off obesity than dying from it. Earnings from books devoted to dieting are counted in the millions. The typical help-yourself book imbues the reader with zealous enthusiasm so that he attempts to alter his life in one fell swoop. Unfortunately, it is impossible to change a lifetime of habits overnight.

The weight-reduction industry grosses billions more with reducing schemes that are for the most part fraudulent or fruitless. In an effort to become slim, we allow ourselves to be hypnotized, psychoanalyzed, and mesmerized. We go on high-caloric diets, low-caloric diets, grapefruit diets, water diets, drinkers diets, crash diets, starvation diets, and sex-substituted diets. We gulp diet pills, snack on diet cookies, guzzle protein drinks, and chomp on diet gum. We try to reduce with belts, with machines, and with wraps; augment the fight with hormones and creams; and, in a last desperate gasp, join diet clubs in order to commiserate about our plight. But the majority of us who attempt the above will emerge in much the same fashion as when we started: overweight.

The type of food that we eat is more important than the amount. There is no such thing as fattening food, only high- and low-caloric food. With respect to gaining or losing body weight, food is characterized by a single parameter—calories, a measure for the amount of food energy we consume. As a unit of measurement, it is unchangeable. If caloric intake exceeds caloric output, the body stores the surplus as fat. This process constitutes an immutable law of physics.

The Only Effective Method for Losing Weight is to reduce the caloric income and, for most of us, any loyally followed diet will produce weight loss. A good reducing regimen should be one that you can live with, and not just for a short time. Most fad diets that drastically restrict your selection of food eventually become so boring that you cannot sustain them for very long. If the reducing program is not comfortable, it won't work. The biggest single mistake in dieting is the belief that there is some miraculous way to lose weight and keep it off without effort. There is no magic. We have inherited a body made to hunt and run, not to sit at a desk, and we consume more energy than we biologically need.

Most of us diet for the wrong reasons: we want to look better, not live longer, and we try to lose weight without honest effort. To be slender and stay that way, one must pay the price of eternal vigilance. The road to slimness is not paved with gadgets, gimmicks, contrivances, crash or fasting diets, special foods or pills. Although fad diets can cause pounds to fade, they dupe us for they do nothing to help the individual learn the right way to lose excess pounds and keep them off. The lasting cure for obesity is the substitution of proper eating and drinking habits for improper ones, which all too often we learned as toddlers.

Weight reduction pills are dangerous, even under a physician's supervision, as the body's metabolism is so accelerated that when the pills are discontinued, profound physiologic symptoms may occur. Reducing creams and the elaborate array of machines, vibrators, massaging belts, wraps, and the like that are ballyhooed rapidly thin one's wallet while fattening the entrepreneur's. For the most part, they are without merit and are promoted by misleading advertisements that prey on the gullibility of the American public.

Starving for a few days may be exhilarating, but it can also be dangerous for your health. Crash diets (I've never seen anything good come from a crash) require such radical changes in eating patterns that they can only add to the physical strain of dieting itself. Besides, the initial pounds shed are mostly water rather than fat so there is no real weight loss at all. This is particularly true in all quick-weight-loss diets. Under ordinary circumstances, carbohydrates supply the greater part of our caloric requirements while fat is burned at a relatively slow rate. Deprived of its principal fuel (carbohydrate), the body is obliged to burn protein instead, producing a physiologic body condition known as ketosis. A dramatic side effect of ketosis is the body's rapid loss of water, which is generally misinterpreted by the dieter as fat loss. Since the body is approximately two-thirds water, within several weeks it is possible to lose a considerable amount of fluid without any reduction in the total body fat.

With dieting, the body initially calls upon glycogen (stored sugar) to provide energy. This glycogen, which is stored in the liver, muscles, and the protein of lean tissue, exists in combination with water. When the glycogen and protein go, so does the water. After the first weeks of any diet, however, weight loss becomes apparent as the glycogen disappears and body energy becomes entirely dependent on fat.

In a simple equation, one pound of fat, added or taken off, equals 3500 calories. If, for instance, you cut down 500 calories a day, this will mean the loss of one pound a week; a 1000-calorie daily deficit, two pounds per week. In addition to cutting calories, if you also burn up an extra 500 calories a day by physical exercise, you will take off an extra pound per week for weight depends not only on caloric intake, but also on how many calories the body burns up in physical activity. It all adds up to a slow but surefire method of losing weight. Over the long run, this loss will be much more likely to stay lost.

In some measure, exercise alone, without caloric restriction, produces weight loss; it also has some advantages over dieting exclusively. First, exercise improves the function of the heart, lungs, and muscular system. Second, it can be an enjoyable leisure-time activity, whereas few people enjoy dieting. Third, the weight shed through exercise consists primarily of fat as opposed to the water loss or loss of vital lean tissue that can occur with crash or fad diets.

Many people, however, fear that increased exercise stimulates an increase in appetite with a consequent food intake that is equal to or greater in energy value than the energy expended. This is not true. Scientific research indicates either no change in food intake with moderate exercise or a slight decrease with vigorous exercise.

Although jogging is quite fashionable today, an easier form of exercise is simply walking and most of us can do that. Walk when you can instead of driving, use steps instead of elevators, walk the dog more often. Those little jaunts can prolong your life.

Actually, most people who diet rarely maintain their weight loss for any length of time. This is due to the fact that the most important factor in *durable* weight loss is the effort the overweight person makes to modify permanently eating habits and his or her self-image. This is a great challenge, especially in a society where advertising agencies are paid enormous sums to make us drool. If this challenge is not met, adipose tissue will progressively accumulate in conspicuous areas of the body such as the abdomen, sides of the thighs, and the buttocks.

The Abdomen

The flabby, protuberant, and pendulous abdomen becomes an aesthetic problem since it cannot be corrected by exercise or any form of weight reduction. Although men occasionally exhibit this, the problem affects more women, especially those who are overweight and have had children.*

When the skin stretches and bulges outward from pregnancy or obesity, stretch marks can form. They resist all present-day "miracle" drugs that are as numerous as they are ineffective. Emollients do not help prevent these marks either, for the fragmenting of elastin and collagen takes place in the deep layers where these protein fibers are stretched beyond their elastic limit and break down. Although the protuberant fat and skin can be removed, stretch marks, although made less obvious, are not

**There is a saying that sorrow dims all beauty and childbearing thickens the sweetest shape.*

removed with surgery; their treatment lies in prevention. The less weight gained, the less chance of stretch marks.

Corsets, binders, and abdominal supports temporarily gather in and pull up the "pot" belly, but they are an inconvenience and over the long haul, are uncomfortable to hide behind. The only effective method to graphically cleanse the abdomen and restore its muscle tone is by an operation known as abdominal lipectomy. Although it is a prolonged dissection, involving repair of the abdominal musculature and relocation of the navel, the public lightly refers to it as the "tummy tuck."

Just a Shave and a Trim Please

The operation takes about two hours and is a hospital procedure performed under a general anesthetic. The patient is prepped and draped to create a sterile field. A horizontal incision that extends from side to side is made just above the pubic hair line. Only the topmost part of the hair is shaved, thereby eliminating the postoperative discomfort associated with its regrowth. Even with the briefest of bikinis, the resulting scar will be hidden.

The dissection is carried upward toward the navel. Since this has also sagged, it must be raised to a higher position. The surgeon frees the navel by making a circular incision around it. He then carries the dissection downward to the belly muscles so that the navel is maintained as a circular island with a stalk of fatty tissue and vessels extending down to the muscles.

The dissection then continues upward around the core supporting the navel to just below the rib cage. After reinforcing the weakened muscles with sutures, the surgeon pulls the abdominal flap downward and removes excess skin and fat. The operating table at this stage is bent in a jackknife position; this allows the maximum amount of tissue to be removed and facilitates closure. The operating table is then straightened and a buttonhole opening is made in the proper position in the abdominal flap through which the umbilical stalk is pulled. The newly reconstructed belly button is sewn into place with fine sutures. The surgeon next closes the horizontal incision completely, inserts drains to remove serum or blood that might accumulate, and applies a large dressing and binder to the area.

The patient is kept in flexion (jackknife position) and at bed rest for forty-eight hours. Deep breathing and leg exercises are carried out to prevent circulatory and lung complications. After two days, the dressing is changed and the drains are removed. The patient is then discharged from the hospital with the standard medications.

Discomfort is moderate and except for the patient's experiencing some difficulty walking for several days, the convalescence presents no problem. Complications are minimal. Blood can collect under the flap, but the drains handle that. If the incision breaks down from excessive tension, thickened scars can certainly result. They can be minimized, however, by cortisone injections.

By the fifth day, the binder is discarded and a waist girdle substituted. The navel sutures are removed at this time. Within fourteen days, all sutures are out, but the patient is advised to wear the girdle for approximately six weeks. Showers are permissible one week after surgery; bathing in two weeks. The patient must avoid strenuous activity and all body exercises for six weeks; appreciable abdominal pain is the penalty if this advice is not heeded. An example of the tummy tuck is illustrated in Figure 9-5.

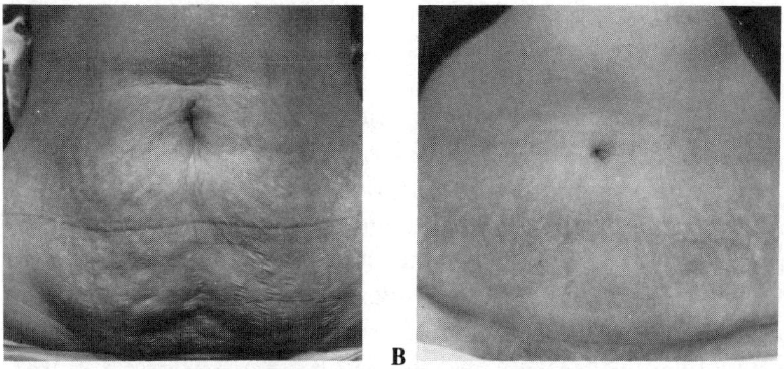

A B

Figure 9-5. A. A 26-year-old with diffuse stretch marks, excess skin, and abdominal sagging following two pregnancies. **B.** Seven months postoperative. Scar is still quite noticeable, but will fade more with time. It is well within the bikini line.

Meet Livia

The psychological and physical benefits of the precedure are typified by this case history:

Livia was a fifty-year-old Caucasian widow. She came in requesting a breast augmentation and corrective work on her abdomen. She was a prominent optometrist who had until recently been passing through life rather than living it. When she was thirty, her husband, mother, and father had been killed in an automobile accident, leaving her with her own child and three much younger sisters and brother. The deaths were the most appalling tragedy she had ever known. It ended her social interest in the real world and she retreated into the past, becoming both mother and father to the surviving brood.

She had become deeply immersed in her work and her role as a parent. In the process, she had neglected herself. Over the years, she had become enormously overweight, but gave it little concern.

In her fiftieth year, she had authored a book on a method of rejuvenating the human lens by the wearing of contact lenses. The concept had an enormous success, requiring promotional, personal and TV appearances. After prolonged discussions with her publisher, she realized that fat, frumpy, and fifty wasn't where it was at. She had gone on a fanatic diet, losing fifty pounds and although she had slimmed, what had slimmed had sagged.

Her initially small breasts had shrunk even smaller and looked like two nipples tacked onto the chest wall, presumably to break up the monotony. The abdominal skin was loose, flabby, and hanging, literally covering over a part of the pubis.

She wanted both procedures at once, but when the risks in doing both simultaneously were explained to her, she relented and allowed the surgeon to dictate the sequence. She was admitted to the hospital and the augmentation was performed. Within ten days she was back and, under general anesthesia, underwent the abdominal lipectomy. As an added bonus, deep internal sutures were placed to narrow her waist. She recovered from this procedure within two weeks. After six weeks, she was ready to begin her promotional tour and it was apparent that this was not brittle enthusiasm. It was also quite obvious that with her remodeled figure she had developed an aura of femininity that she had lacked before.

Out, Out Damned Fat

Excess fat also accumulates along the sides of the thighs and around the buttocks. There is more fat in the thigh and buttock areas of most women, an anatomical fact which imbues the female with her shapely contours. Unfortunately, this fat can lead to unsightly deposits as women age and it is not readily lost with the usual diets and exercise.

When the thighs or buttocks are squeezed or pinched between the hands, this produces dimples, bulges, and deformations (the mattress and orange peel phenomena) which, unfortunately, are viewed by some as the cardinal signs of an invented disease with a coined name—cellulite. The phenomena are actually sex-typical features of the skin of the thighs and buttocks of most women and a natural consequence of aging, not a sign of disease. There is a familial tendency to develop this; the condition is often combined with obesity, but can also appear in slim-waisted females.

So-called cellulite is a cosmetic defect that obsesses and tortures millions of women from adolescence to senescence. This manufactured "disease" is a normal abnormality, but it has spawned a billion-dollar industry of lay aestheticians and legitimate physicians who offer futile treatment yet boast of numerous successes.

The treatment of cellulite has given life to those "beauty parlors" using salves, creams and, in particular, body wrapping as a method to rub out this "ugly fat." The concept of "spot reduction" rests on the widely held belief that by exercising a specific body area with devices such as wraps, belts, and vibrators, the fat in that part will be reduced. The individual is usually wrapped with sheets impregnated with a salt solution ($MgSO_4$—Epsom salt). This is supposed to induce local perspiration, flush toxins from the body, and break up the lumpy fat. It does squeeze out some body water and it is this loss that provides the apparent reduction. However, this effect vanishes as the tissues are replenished with fluid. Practitioners of these treatments do not know, or perhaps fail to mention to their clients, that fat is fat. You can't move it from one place to another; you can't break it up by wrapping, vibrating or pounding. At best, these methods may be a psychological crutch to encourage people to stay on their diet and exercise. But there is absolutely no scientific evidence to show that by themselves, spot reducers, vibrators, or any of the various types of body wraps alter the metabolism of fat.

The injection of spreading enzymes as promoted by French physicians, "rice" treatments, electrophysical methods, and the application of salves or suppositories are no more effective than placebo therapy.

The most important factor in the treatment is prevention—the avoidance of overweight from childhood on. Obesity starting in the teens is apt to be more solid and immovable than weight acquired in later years. In adults, conservative treatment for this fat is by diet, massage, and exercise. Usual exercises won't do it and those directed toward a particular portion of the body such as hips or abdomen won't be effective unless performed vigorously. Very effective are straight leg kicks executed in thigh-deep water, running in soft sand, bike riding, and karate. Massaging with the hand or a brush is beneficial. The massage should always be directed away from the periphery toward the heart. This also tends to improve the circulation of the blood and lymph, and is helpful to women with vascular problems of the legs.

Surgical Procedures

If conservative measures do not help you, the cold blade will. However, thigh and buttock surgery create some of the least attractive scars generated by cosmetic surgery.

Formerly, to correct loose, bulging skin of the inner part of the thigh, an incision was usually made parallel to the crease of the groin. Experience revealed that these scars moved downward with

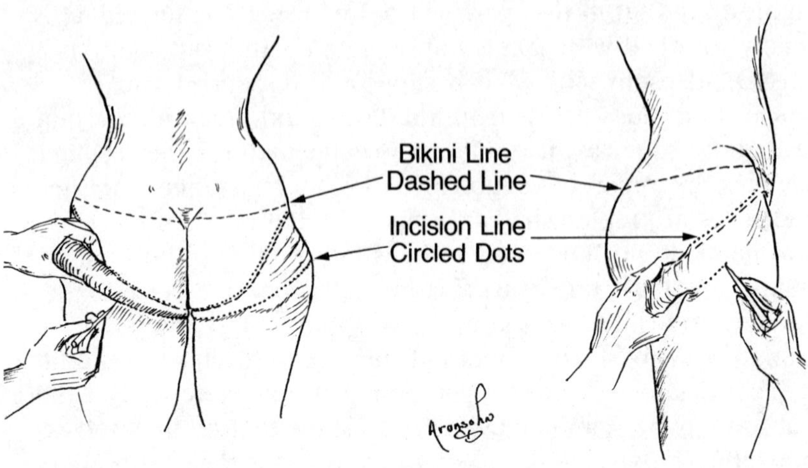

Figure 9-6 The amount of tissue to be resected is measured with the patient in the upright position. The lowermost incision is brought up to the superior line which is within the bikini line and thus covered by it.

time so as to be visible with the usual bathing apparel. Cutting along the inside of the leg from groin to kneecap will remove the problem, but few patients are willing to accept the permanent, visible scars. Therefore, surgeons usually make the incisions in the deep groin area and carry them upward above the groin toward the outer portion of the lower abdomen. In the back, the incision curves around the buttock fold. The surgeon separates the skin from the underlying tissue, lifts it upward, and removes the excess skin and fat. In the front, the flap is then sutured at this higher abdominal position. Conventional swimsuits will hide the scars.

The excess accumulation of fat in women's outer hips causes a characteristic deformity that resembles riding breeches and is accordingly given this name. Here again, a vertical incision along the outer thigh will remedy this but will leave prominent, visible scars. The best approach for removal is with a crescent-shaped excision of skin and fat that extends along the buttock fold in back and curves along each outer thigh toward the hip bone (Figure 9-6). The removal of excess fat and skin along this curve trims the hips and lifts the buttocks. Resulting scars are hidden by brief pants (Figure 9-7).

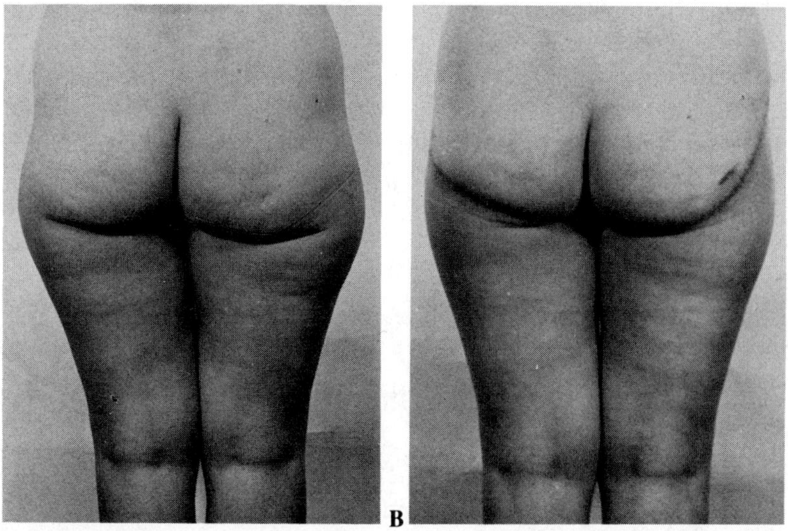

A B

Figure 9-7 A. Bulging thighs and sagging buttocks. **B.** Subtle, but more graceful curve to thighs and buttocks. They are firmer and more elevated—four months postoperative.

As in the abdominal lipectomy, planning of the incisions in these surgeries is extremely important in achieving the desired results. The surgeries are performed in the hospital under a general anesthetic, require several hours of operating time followed by bandaging from abdomen to thighs. For several days the patient remains in a semiflexed position while in bed, and is restricted to a low residue diet. She is discharged by the fourth day and sutures are gradually removed in stages from the eighth to the fourteenth day. The convalescense is approximately two weeks, but vigorous exercise is prohibited for about six weeks.

Surgeons have also removed fat from the sides of the thighs via a small incision through which they introduced a long curette and scraped the fat away. Not only was this procedure very tedious, but on occasion some morsels of amputated fat were left behind. The loose, floating fat subsequently gave rise to fluid accumulations and to unsightly irregular skin surfaces. A suction-curette instrument has now been invented that not only removes the unwanted fat, but also suctions it away and prevents the detached tissue from being lost. To date, it has shown promise in removing large amounts of fat through a small stab incision that requires minimal postoperative care and leaves an insignificant scar.

Although there have been tremendous strides made in breast augmentation, little attention has been given to techniques for enlarging the buttocks of people with flat derrieres. Although the literature mainly deals with reducing this area, silicone implant augmentations are feasible. Patients must be highly motivated, however, since minimal pressure can be put on this area for a week to ten days and the operation involves a prolonged hospitalization.

The surgical fee for an abdominal lipectomy is approximately $4000 and is usually defrayed by insurance. Inner- and outer-thigh procedures run about $2500 and are not usually covered by insurance. Tightening and raising the buttock can also touch the $3000 mark.

The surgical fee for breast augmentation can range from $2000 to $3000, and is usually not covered by insurance. For bilateral breast reduction, the surgical fee may vary from $3000 to $4000. As this procedure is considered physiological in nature, it is covered by insurance. As in all general anesthesias, there is also an anesthetist's fee, which is exclusive of the surgical cost.

Elbows, Hands, and Bat Wings

Another problem caused by excess fat, gravity, and age is the hanging skin that droops from the undersurface of the upper arms. This pathology is known as the "bat wing" deformity and presents a problem in its repair. By the use of a sinuous incision from armpit to elbow, the excess skin and fat can be removed. Compression bandages are worn for several days and all sutures are removed within two weeks. For several weeks there will be swelling in the area that may even extend to the hands. This type of incision breaks up the continuous scar, making it less evident. The patient, however, must be made aware that no matter what technique is employed, there will be a visible scar as no camouflage points exist throughout this area.

Any fly-by-night can correct bat wing deformities, but it is best left to surgical experts, whose prices range from $1500 to $2000.

Elbows and hands present specific problems. The wrinkles along the elbow joint come and go with bending and straightening the arm. They are not amenable to any surgical, peeling, or abrading process and are better left alone. With aging, fat can disappear from the back of the hands, exaggerating the prominent veins that may be present. Droplets of silicone judiciously injected between the veins can plump up the hands and give them a more youthful look. The veins can also be stripped away much as one would for varicose veins in the legs. Because of the swelling and bruising that occur, only several veins at a time can be removed, making the process long and drawn out. Freckles and pigmentations of the hands are readily peeled away, but will return if the hands are continually exposed to the sun. In theory, cutting away loose, wrinkled skin from the back of the hands makes sense; in practice, it is a procedure which gives a less than satisfactory cosmetic result and yields a very visible scar. It is not recommended. To apply a powerful caustic to the back of the hands in an attempt to tighten wrinkled skin is dangerous, because the hands are not enriched with the regenerating units that exist in the face. This is also not advised as severe scarring may occur.

You've Come A Long Way, Baby

Just about 100 years ago, the bodies of women were bound by corsets and convention. The corset molded women's forms into the famous "hourglass" figure. Convention prohibited exhibiting any part of it.

It took a twentieth-century world to strip away the heretofore well-covered skin of mature women. The trend of today's liberated woman is to uncover more of her torso. Since the slim female figure is in vogue in contemporary society, this moral striptease has sparked an increased interest in torso touch-ups.

If, sometimes through genetic accidents, the body turns out badly constructed, the cosmetic surgeon can help. If the aged body needs rearranging, the cosmetic surgeon can help. Responding to society's mania for self-improvement, he can flatten, raise or tuck in any part of the torso. All that's required is a push in the right direction.

Q&A

When is the best time to have breast augmentation?

Breast enlargement can be performed when full development of the breast has been attained, at about twenty years of age. However, if you plan to have children, it might be wise to defer the operation until you have your brood as the pregnancies will adversely alter the shape of the breast with or without an implant.

What will happen if I get pregnant after a "tummy tuck"?

Chances are you'll have a baby. There's even a better chance that the pregnancy will undo what the surgery accomplished. If you anticipate more children, pass on the abdominal operation until you have had your family.

Will my breasts feel natural and have the same sensation after augmentation?

For all practical purposes, the breasts following enlargement will feel normal to the touch. If the implant has been inserted through the nipple site, sensation may be dulled for several weeks because of injury to the small nerves, but will return as healing takes place.

My breasts are sagging but not pendulous. What can be done for them?

Here, an increase in breast size without correction of the sagging would result in an unattractive bosom. A reconstruction must be carried out to firm up the breasts and at the same time implants are inserted to give them fullness and extra thrust. The scars are similar to those resulting from the correction of a large, slumping breast.

What is the best way to lose weight?

There is no mystery to the mechanism of weight gain or loss—you gain when the caloric intake exceeds the caloric amount expended. Any nutritionally sound, well-balanced slimming regimen that can be followed throughout life will produce weight loss. Crash diets, fasting diets, fad diets of any sort can be dangerous and encourage poor eating habits. Remember, the goal of any practical, long-term dietary plan is to learn to live with food, not without it.

What is this new suction procedure that is being used for the removal of "Cellulite" and localized fat deposits?

This technique is called "LIPOLYSIS" and is remarkable because of the small incision (about one-half inch in length) and the minimal time of postoperative disability. The technique was developed and perfected in France and has been used there since 1977. It is based on the injection of a saline solution into the fat deposits, usually under general anesthesia. The temporarily loosened fat is then removed by suction via the incision. With "LIPOLYSIS", normal body curves and contours can be improved and scarring held to a minimum. Each incision is closed with only one stitch that is self-dissolving.

The localized fat deposits that respond to this technique are on thighs, hips, buttocks, knees, arms, abdomen and underneath the chin – areas which are unresponsive to dieting and exercise.

Postoperative pain is mild and readily responds to the usual analgesics. Small suction drains are maintained for 24 hours after surgery. Elastic bandages applied after surgery are removed on the seventh day. Light massage of the operated areas is begun on the tenth day. Full exercise on the fourteenth postoperative day is mandatory in order to minimize adhesion formation between the skin and the underlying tissues. Although results can usually be seen immediately after surgery (even with the dressings in place), complete healing is not expected for three months or more.

[illegible]

[illegible]

There's no mystery to the [illegible]

[illegible]

10

Cosmetics, Massages, and Facials: Promises, Promises, Promises

To most women, whether they are socialites, career women, or housewives, cosmetics are psychologically important. Most of them know that there's no need to have classic features in order to be beautiful. They understand that it is the overall facial arrangement and its particular harmony that can impart the impression of beauty. And they are aware that the skillful application of makeup produces an artistic enhancement as they highlight their good features and shade out the bad.

Actually the cosmetic industry is an industry founded on promises. It promises that it can help you look glamorous. It promises that some of its compounds will even make you look younger. Some of their products promise that they can remove wrinkles and make your skin smoother and satinlike. The cosmetic industry promises that its products are safe enough for a baby's skin.

For the most part, cosmetics do help the skin look better and some even make you feel good. But much of what their manufacturers lead you to expect in the whipped-cream-and-meringue women's magazines never comes to pass, but they say any lackluster performance of their product is due to your inadequacy, not the cosmetic's. Most commercial skin preparations are of greater psychological value than real benefit.

Compared with food and drugs, cosmetics are relatively immune from governmental regulation and although cosmetics today are reputed to be thoroughly tested and harmless, notable exceptions occur. For example, many hair dyes contain "coal-tar" derivatives that are known to cause cancer. Numerous cosmetics contain irritants that have so sensitized some patients that they have needed medical attention. More than a few have required hospitalization.

Because the cosmetic manufacturers jealously guard their trade secrets, they are not compelled to print complete ingredient information on the labels of their products. The woman with sensitive skin, therefore, should be quite cautious in purchasing any cosmetic and should follow two basic guidelines: be wary of overstated claims and stop using any cosmetic or other product that causes any type of allergic reaction.

Most women buy too many cosmetics and just as many misapply them. Cosmetics should be used to hide, enhance, or dramatize features. Besides covering skin blemishes, makeup correctly applied can repaint the canvas of the face to improve the portrait that others see.

Cosmetics can change the shape of the eyes and enhance their glow; they can make thin lips seem fuller or, if need be, full ones thinner. With the proper shades, a nose slightly askew can look straighter and a wide bridge appear narrower. Cheekbones will seem higher with strategic highlights, although, of course, they can attain prominence permanently by silicone implants or by the injection of silicone fluid. Eyebrows are the only aspect of the face that make-up can revamp in many ways. They can be arched, raised or lowered, made thin or full, and are easily altered to compensate for aesthetic eye deficiencies.

Figment, Fiction, and Fantasy

Despite their glittering claims, cosmetics cannot nourish your skin. Emollients can lubricate, soften, and preserve the epidermal layers. They can also minimize chapping and windburn, but they cannot literally feed the skin from the outside as nourishment derives from the bloodstream, not the skin surface. Skin is a naturally impervious barrier and very little can cross the intact layer. Certain hormone and cortisone creams can penetrate the skin, but these come under Food and Drug Administration (FDA) scrutiny, and are labeled as drugs, not cosmetics. They are obtainable only by prescription.

Cosmetics cannot permanently clog pores. The basic reason is that the pore, which is really the opening of a hair follicle, cannot be clogged from without unless, of course, the cosmetic is put on with a trowel. Any grease content of a pore comes from the natural change within the skin, not from any surface application.

Cosmetic cleansing creams, despite their promoters' claims, cannot clean extra deep and are no more effective in cleaning the skin than conventional methods. Extra-deep cleansing is impossible because *all* cleaning can only affect the surface layers of the skin. What about facial saunas as a facial cleanser? Sauna-induced perspiration does rid the face of surface dirt but, as a facial cleanser, is no more effective than the usual methods. Also, any temperature extreme—too hot or too cold—can be drying. A steaming hot tub may be great for your aching bones and sore muscles, but lukewarm water is better for your skin. As we become older, there is a loss and degeneration of the elastic tissue which surrounds blood vessels. Heat makes these vessels swell, thereby stretching and straining the tissue. The less tension on this elastic tissue, the longer it will last and the fewer broken capillaries we'll notice on our faces.

No cosmetic preparation rubbed into the skin will permanently reduce major wrinkles caused by aging since no commercial product exists that can restore the skin's thickness and elasticity. At best, emollients and moisturizers can temporarily de-emphasize some fine lines around the eyes and mouth. Nevertheless, there are various skin preparations on the market that claim to do this. There are also many advertised exercise and massage programs that make these unwarranted claims.

A cleansing sponge, such as Buf-Puf®, can minimize wrinkles by invigorating the skin. The face is thoroughly scrubbed for approximately one minute with this sponge, with or without soap added. The sponge removes any surface cells that are present and creates a mild, intentional irritation that produces facial swelling. This plumps up the skin between the pores, making them appear smaller while obscuring the fine lines around the eyes. The scrubbing can be repeated daily as long as the face shows no intense inflammation.

Small glabellar frowns (those between the eyebrows) can also be concealed with a device using the same idea. "Frownies," which contain an acetate backing, produce a localized irritation when applied to the skin. This mild reaction causes swelling of the skin that fills out the lines. The ends of the Frownies should be cut (feathered) where they meet the skin for when they are left on overnight, in the morning there may be a sharp ridge at the skin-frownie junction.

Moisturizers' claim to fame is their ability to rehydrate the skin and keep up its water content. A much better and less expensive way to achieve this is by drinking more water. Dry skin is caused by a lack of water, not a lack of oil. Most of us do not take in enough daily fluid, a serious oversight as it is important for good health. As we age, it is even more important because the water-binding capacity of the cells is reduced leading to increased dryness of the skin.

Your skin also becomes dry when you wash your face with soap and water for these cleanse away the skin's natural film of oil that retards water evaporation. Don't be misled by advertising about super-fatted or fat-added soaps. Manufacturers claim that these soaps thoroughly cleanse the face and still leave an adequate film of oil behind to lubricate and moisturize the skin. No soap can remove oil and simultaneously add oil. Washing with *any kind* of soap removes the natural oils from the skin surface.

Stripped of this protective oily coat, the skin loses water to the air. Where the climate is arid and the humidity low, water evaporation is extremely rapid, leading to dry, lined, and wrinkled skin.

Emollients are skin protectants because their fatty compounds make the skin soft and pliable while mechanically trapping water in the skin surface. There are many expensive perfumed emollients that line the shelves of beauty shops; as good as any is pure petroleum jelly (Vaseline®), which should be lightly smeared over the face, hands, feet, and elbows sometime before retiring—otherwise one just slithers off the bed.

Facial Exercises: Don't Stretch It

Many patients inquire about facial exercises and ask what are the best kinds to maintain facial tone. Countless books and classes are available on this subject, all of them by lay people who claim that sag, wrinkles, lines, and dark circles can be erased by making "funny faces." Undeterred by their ignorance, the advocates of facial exercise stand on the premise that a "muscle is a muscle; so the muscles of the face must be toned just like the muscles of the body."

Facial exercises are not beneficial; indeed, they are *harmful* for they promote lines and wrinkles. The concept of facial exercise to maintain muscle tone to prevent sagging of the facial skin is an erroneous one.

First of all, when the skin begins to wrinkle, it is less firmly connected to the underlying muscles and the skin envelope has now become too big. Secondly, the surface muscles of the face differ from those of the body in that the former are attached intimately to the skin and control its movements. Contraction of the facial muscles pulls the skin, which adapts by forming lines or folds at right angles to the direction of muscle pull. Because of this direct attachment, the skin is moved by the slightest activation of these muscles, thus permitting an eloquent repertoire of facial expression.

In the body, muscles originate on and attach to bone, controlling the movement of the bone, which in turn produces body motion. Only in the face can muscle contraction move skin. Contraction of body muscles obviously requires greater energy than contraction of facial muscles where only skin movements are involved.

In the absence of any paralysis or muscle damage to the face, muscle tone is continually in effect and is constantly challenged by natural facial expressions such as talking, smiling, laughing, and crying. Body muscles, however, will weaken and atrophy if unused for prolonged periods. Thus, we become weak after extended bed rest (even though we may not be ill). Assuming proper nutrition, exercise can and does strengthen these muscles by causing them to enlarge. The stronger the muscle, the more power and energy potential it possesses. Facial muscles, on the other hand, require a minimum of energy to exert their action and call for no such exercise.

Some proponents of facial exercise claim that wrinkles and lines form because the muscles are used in only one direction. What these people fail to understand, or are apparently unaware of, is that all muscles are so constructed that pull is possible in only one direction—from the point of attachment (origin) toward the point of insertion. Since this pull cannot be reversed, the lines formed by contraction of facial muscles cannot be counteracted by grimacing, sneering, or any other idiotic contortions known as facial exercises. Endeavoring to do so is like trying to restore the tread on an automobile tire by driving the car backwards. *All* driving wears the tread. *All* vigorous facial movements encourage lines and wrinkles. The face is like a piece of machinery—the less you use it, the longer it is going to last and the nicer it will look.

Yet some people claim that facial exercises seem to help. These individuals are probably blessed with a youthful genetic make-up. They are also careful of their weight and of sun exposure. *Initially*, they have minimal sag and few wrinkles or lines. Nor will they develop these aging defects as rapidly as others not so genetically blessed. Their facial tone is more apt to remain vibrant with aging, but since they utilize facial exercises, that youthful look is attributed to the exercises and from their viewpoint, they work.

Individuals who sustain a one-sided facial paralysis (especially at an early age) exhibit few lines on the paralyzed side, whereas the opposite side of the face develops lines and creases in marked contrast. In fact, this observation led to a cosmetic surgical procedure wherein the nerve to a facial muscle was severed to eradicate the lines or frown that the muscles caused. Thus we have dramatic illustration that the less the facial muscles are used, the less lined the face.

Massages, Masks, and Midlife. Aye, There's the Rub

Patients relate how great it is to have a facial massage. Do they help the skin? The benefits of facial massage, if any, are slight and primarily for the psyche. Without going into the many causes of skin degeneration, there is a loss of skin elasticity and with the ever-present forces of gravity, the skin and fat of the face sag. The regions involved are the nasolabial folds, the cheeks, the jawline (the jowls), and the neck. In these areas, the fat is not fixed to bone and is easily displaced by gravity, loss of elasticity, and manipulation—an important argument against facial massage. A facial massage may temporarily improve skin circulation, but the danger of displacing fat far outweighs any benefit it might yield. Facial massages are not recommended. Body massages, on the other hand, are beneficial.

Facial masks also add very little and their effect is mainly psychological. As the mask dries, it tightens and pulls the skin, so the user thinks that something must be happening. When the mask is rinsed off, surface skin is removed along with surface debris—the skin feels cleaner and looks fresher. However, in any realistic long-term sense, it won't make any difference if you use facials or not—they don't cure crow's feet or blemishes, and they won't prevent you from aging.

There are many fancy, high-priced facial masks on the market. The following is one that performs as well as any commercially packaged product: mix one egg white with one teaspoon of honey. Smooth this mixture over your entire face allowing a wide margin for the lids. Leave on for fifteen minutes and wash off with warm water followed by a cool rinse. Once a week is okay.

There are many other homemade beauty preparations that temporarily freshen, cleanse, or tighten the skin. They range from cucumbers to strawberries, blended or intact, and are well documented in natural-beauty books and therefore will not be belabored on these pages. Here again, what is reputed to have worked well for a movie siren or other famous woman may not necessarily work as well for you.

Do facial stimulators work? If there has been trauma or nerve injury to the facial muscles and they are not functioning properly, galvanic facial exercisers are helpful as the electric current stimulates the muscle which moves the skin. In this manner, the muscle will not atrophy from disuse nor will the face sag while the nerve or muscle is recovering. In the absence of any nerve or muscle injury, they serve no useful purpose.

The constant use of false eyelashes or strip lashes together with aging take their toll on the natural lash. The less they are used, the longer the natural lashes will last. Reserve them only for special occasions.

What the public should completely understand is that no preparation or device applied to the face can ever replace moderate living, proper nutrition, adequate rest, and the ability to cope with stress. Both natural and synthetic products are promoted as capable of performing miracles; the reader should make his or her own decision regarding these claims.

By the time we reach fifty, most of us have the face we deserve. Other than the fortunate inheritance of youthful genes, the best way to appear ageless is to stay slim, avoid the sun, and refrain from smoking. Those who follow that advice will not have to lie about their age; their skin will do it for them.

We already know why it is better to be thin than fat. The danger from too much sunning is not so well known. Tanning is the reaction of the skin to an insidious but deadly assault as sunlight carves up your face little by little with prolonged exposure. By the way, the sun's rays cannot penetrate glass installed in homes or cars. These are made from silica that actinic rays (those producing chemical change) cannot cross. Infrared (heat) rays do travel through silica and will make you warm, but it is impossible to acquire a tan through ordinary glass. A variety of quartz glass is the primary medium in sun lamps.

As for smoking, unless you decide to quit, your problem isn't going to be smoking—your problem is going to be staying alive. Smoking not only kills you early, but while you're managing to stay alive, it can also age you quicker than need be. Nicotine is a vasoconstrictor that causes the blood vessels to narrow, decreasing blood flow and nourishment to the skin. Blood hemoglobin has a greater affinity for carbon monoxide (which is in the smoke inhaled) than for oxygen and rapidly combines with it to form carboxy-hemoglobin. This displacement of blood oxygen (oxyhemoglobin) by the poisonous carbon monoxide robs the tissue cells of oxidation and adversely affects their nourishment. Thus deprived, the skin will not only appear sallow, but will also age and develop wrinkles at a faster pace.

After a woman's face, her breasts attract the most attention. Innumerable procedures are advocated for building up the breasts, ranging from exercises, manipulation, and massages, to devices that claim to enlarge them. Without exception, all such procedures are useless. The breast contains no muscles except for the smooth muscle in the nipple and is made up primarily of fatty and glandular tissue. The circumferential chest measurement will increase as the back and chest muscles expand in size with exercises prescribed in such programs. But no increase in cup size will occur as fat and glandular tissue do not enlarge with any kind of exercise.

Normal support of the breast is supplied by the breast ligaments and the skin envelope. Wearing a bra relieves tension of the skin and ligaments and therefore can minimize sagging. A bra should be worn during the day.

The Bottom Line

It is amazing how much quackery still exists in a society that has left its footprints on the moon. So often things are introduced in the cosmetic and health-aid industry which have no basis in fact. We spend billions each year on products that are a complete waste. There is a segment of the population who, either through ignorance, panic, or desperation will grasp at any agent that offers them relief for whatever their ill may be. Not that they need or want to be hoodwinked, but it is a psychological quirk in all of us—hope springs eternal—that makes us do the irrational things we do.

Cosmetics easily slip into the above category if everything their makers claim were believed. But whether their claims are credible or deceptive, cosmetics are here to stay. They will continue to be very expensive to the consumer even though they are actually cheap to produce. There is a logical reason for all this. Psychological pricing is part of their sales appeal for a prestige product that promises a fantasy must have a fantastic price—what the cosmetic industry really sells is hopes, dreams, and moonbeams.

It is a $15 billion-dollar-a-year moonbeam which annually increases about 10 percent despite economic boom or recession. Every day this multi-billion-dollar beauty business tells every woman she could be prettier than she is. Cosmetics commercials make up the single largest category of TV advertising, occupying about 20 percent of all commercial time and they are the main staple of women's popular magazines, in whose pages seldom is heard a discouraging word.

No matter—for regardless of what a particular cosmetic or cream will or will not do, whether they will be costly or just plain expensive, or whether natural or synthetic, most women will continue to use them. To most, the caressing and stroking in applying the cosmetics are a pleasurable expenditure of time and energy and a moment to be with one's own thoughts. With this vast array of artificial products to work from, a genuinely beautiful facial mirage can seemingly materialize.

Q&A

Can cosmetics help delay the aging process?

Some cosmetics, particularly emollients, can check the premature onset of wrinkles by maintaining a supple skin and by minimizing the skin's water loss, but by and large most cosmetics are designed to enhance, camouflage, or beautify the skin and features. They have virtually no rejuvenating or antiaging functions.

What can I tell my young daughter who is just beginning to use cosmetics?

Tell her to KISS her face—Keep It Simple, Sis. Clean hair, clean face, with the minimum of cosmetics to highlight and brighten the features.

If a woman could only use one cosmetic, what would you tell her to buy?

Lipstick. The lure of comely lips has been recognized for ages and they are a very visible sexual signaling device. Lipstick also embodies an emollient action, reducing the incidence of chapped lips.

What is the best way to add moisture to my face?

Drink more water—at least six to eight glasses of water a day, in addition to any other fluids you may take in.

Are facial massages beneficial?

From a gratification standpoint, an individual may derive great pleasure from having a facial massage. In reality, deep, repeated facial massaging causes irreparable harm to the tissues and accelerates the aging process.

11
What Does Tomorrow Hold for Us?

Peering into the future can be a nebulous undertaking, one generally left to parapsychologists and psychics. However, one need not be clairvoyant to see what looms ahead—just glance at the timetable. More scientific and technological advances have been made in the last thirty years than in all the years of recorded medical history. Startling new discoveries will continue at an even swifter pace.

What was possible has been done and what is improbable will be done, for today we are at the cutting edge of an exhilarating future. We have cracked the genetic code and genetic engineering has already begun. Many worry how society will cope with the wonders and terrors of transforming itself. Despite the public's alarm about the possible moral, ethical, and social perils of gene splicing, its vast potential for good is overwhelming.* Genetic human duplication (cloning) is under intense investigation and scientists are at the starting gate champing at the bit. Transplantation and implantation are becoming routine. Healthy test-tube babies have already been born and suddenly we are trembling on the threshold of a new concept in creation.

At present, mankind breeds randomly and promiscuously—a genetic roulette without much regard for the next generation. No expert in animal husbandry would think of tolerating such a casual system. Reproduction in the distant future will be more controlled. We are at the fringe of a new frontier in procreation with the capability of correcting baffling hereditary diseases using a genetic scalpel. I do not think we are light years away from taking advantage of these dramatic breakthroughs.

While we are earthbound, there is little the future promises to prevent the gravitational changes that take place within all of us.

* *Most scientific revolutions, from the observation that the earth was round and circled the sun to the splitting of the atom, evoked the cry of heresy.*

Extraterrestrial travel and space-station living will dramatically change that. The zero gravity of outer space will be reflected in a minimal gravitational pull on our faces and bodies, producing less sag as we age. Although our muscles may experience some initial atrophy, our systems will be able to compensate with isometric exercises and adapt with the help of space medicine.

Because of the rejection mechanism, we still cannot successfully transfer hair from one person to another. However, we may not need to, for male-pattern-baldness may be on the way out. The male hormone, testosterone, is altered through an enzymatic process to dihydrotestosterone, which is the specific hormone identified as causing hair loss. Work is in progress perfecting a technique that will block this enzymatic reaction, that is, hinder the hormone's balding trait without producing any feminizing effect or alteration in male characteristics.

Lasers, cryosurgery, and surgical adhesives for wound closure will all take the sting out of surgery and suture removal. Cosmetic lasers will readily remove tattoos, for the dark areas absorb laser light while the lighter skin remains unaffected. Pulse lasers (interrupted coherent light) have shown great promise in removing port-wine birthmarks that can so disfigure the face. Just as the scalpel replaced the sword, so will the laser and cryosurgery replace the scalpel in many cosmetic and reconstruction procedures. Could not lasers be so controlled that they might be able to alter cartilage to the form we wanted? At present, lasers and cryosurgery permit rapid operating with precision and control. There is a lack of bleeding and little postoperative inflammation, swelling, or pain; the rapid healing results in a minimal scar. Smaller, more practical, and more economical instruments are being developed that will ensure the increased use of these innovative techniques in the future.

We will be stuck with surgical adhesives instead of sutures for the experimental use of adhesives promises that they indeed have a future in operative wound closure. Both hypothermic and hypotensive surgery (see Glossary) will become more routine, making complex surgeries less complicated and allowing a cleaner surgical field for the surgeon.

Without a doubt we will be performing more operations on an older human body. The alchemist's goal has been to turn lead into gold and man's dream has been to achieve eternal youth. The alchemist's dream has become a reality and eternal youth may be a possibility. It is conceivable that humanity's quest for the biblical promise of 120 years of life may yet be attained.

Man may not be as old as his arteries, but he certainly is as sick as his arteries. Much illness today is willful in the sense that it not only results from genetic defects, stress and tissue allergy (rather than age itself), but also from the foolish living habits of people who know better. New techniques and new remedies in medicine and surgery are continually being developed in an effort to extend life. It seems sensible for each of us also to make a special effort in that direction. We eat too much, we smoke too much, we drink too much. This indulging has a deleterious effect on our body—a body that is actually programmed to last much longer than it does. In the future, the proper care and maintenance of ourselves will be incorporated into the school curriculum at a very early age and will be as fundamental as learning the ABCs.

A Hint of Immortality

As stated in chapter 4, cellular therapy to extend the life span has been based mainly on testimonials. Most researchers discount cell-therapy treatments on the grounds that no scientifically controlled studies have ever been carried out to support their effectiveness. Procaine, both ingested and injected (Gerovital therapy), has also been heatedly touted as a rejuvenating drug. The controversy concerning it does not seem to be cooling down, mainly because Gerovital has received some investigative study in the United States.

Many people became aware that taking Gerovital for prolonged periods appeared to enhance their psychic well-being, increase their physical vigor, and improve their looks. Enthusiastic proponents stated that Gerovital reduced the biological age of those treated with it below their chronological age. In simpler terms, this meant that the drug made patients look younger than they actually were—no modest claim. Why did procaine, a standard analgesic, and the integral part of Gerovital, seemingly produce this miraculous result? The key to the mystery was that procaine was found to be a powerful inhibitor of monoamine oxidase. Monoamine oxidase is an enzyme that increases in all aging animals and occurs as a general biological phenomenon. Monoamine oxidase is widely distributed throughout the human body, especially in the central nervous system and as we grow older, its concentration increases. High levels of this enzyme have been found to be related to depression, which is the commonest psychiatric problem of the aged. Consequently, it seemed reasonable that any drug that might curb depression might also be an antiaging factor.

Since oxidase promotes an oxidation reaction, inhibiting this reaction went hand in hand with the "free radical" theory of aging. Free radicals are fragments of molecules with a high electrical charge and cause adverse changes in the body by their oxidizing properties. Antioxidents, or oxidase inhibitors, supposedly deactivate the free radicals, thereby retarding the aging process.

But does Gerovital prolong life? It is difficult to ascertain whether or not it increases the life span of an individual since it is difficult to tell how long a person would live without it and at present no exact biometric age index is available. Research into this controversial drug is continuing.

We are aware that lowering the body temperature adds years to human life. Restricting the diet delays maturity in the young, rejuvenates the immune system in middle age, and increases longevity. But we are now approaching a new period in our understanding of sickness, aging, and death. Scientists are beginning to unlock the secrets of the fundamental component of all living things—the human cell. As cells malfunction, people become ill and as cells deteriorate, people die. Undoubtedly, by the year 2000, two killers, cardiovascular disease and cancer, will be conquered, adding years to life*. A true elixir of youth has yet to be found, and quite possibly will never be, for nature has a way of killing anything that lives. However, a number of interesting and speculative theories are under investigation in experimental laboratories throughout the world whereby the aging process may eventually be controlled. In time, one of these theories may prove correct. When that time comes, aging control will become as vital an issue as birth control.

Have I Got a Part for You

Our lengthened life span will unquestionably add to the

**The common impression that modern medical triumphs have lengthened the human lifespan is not supported by either vital statistics or biologic evidence. Life expectation has increased but our lifespan has remained essentially unchanged since recorded history. Medical advances have simply allowed more people to reach the limit of that fixed lifespan.*

demands for cosmetic surgery. There will be an increased market for organ transplantation and implantation and the future of these techniques is guaranteed. The transplantation of organs from one person to another, in full flow several years ago, has slowed to a trickle. This is because of the rejection that occurred despite the immuno-suppressive drugs used to combat attacking antibodies formed when the body is subjected to a foreign substance, especially protein. Nature devised this immune mechanism largely to protect higher animals against invasion by parasites, bacteria, and viruses, but the defense works equally well against tissues from other higher animals, including those from another person (except an identical twin).

This problem will be solved as work continues. At present, a person's body tissue can be classified just as blood can be classified by type. Transplant "banks" are being set up to serve as clearing houses and to bring potential donors and recipients together on the basis of their tissue type and thus enhance the chances of success.

In the future, surgical scientists will prepare humans for organ transplantation while still within the womb. It is in the foetal stage that life is unable to recognize or reject foreign substances. Various tissue antigens as well as blood-type antigens can be injected into the womb's amniotic fluid to be incorporated by the fetus, allowing that individual to become a universal donor or recipient.

We may not be capable of building a $6 million man, but we are able to replace almost every part in the human body. The body will soon be viewed as a biologic machine requiring spare-part replacement with age and use. What began as a trickle of spare parts for humans has surged to a deluge for surgical implantation, once an exotic procedure, is now routine. Initially developed for medical purposes such as heart valves, artificial lenses, pacemakers, and total hip replacements, implants are filling an increasing consumer need in cosmetic operations on chins, noses, ears, cheeks, and breasts. Aesthetically they are acceptable, and will continue to look even better as refinement continues. However, one of the biggest problems with both transplantation and implantation, indeed with all of medicine and surgery today, is the product-liability fever that has swept this country for the last several years. Malpractice suits and insurance premiums for physician protection are all skyrocketing.

Maybe We Can Work Something Out

There is probably no such thing as a risk-free society, but the trend in medicine is frightening. There is a tendency in this country for people to sue somebody for even the smallest slight or injury. This may be due to the public's awareness that juries too often are overly generous. Also, the lure of a windfall held out by an attorney often proves irresistible, and publicity given to big awards awakens greed that also stimulates lawsuits. Lawyers and plaintiffs presume that juries don't care how much of someone else's money they award, for they are convinced that none of the money will come from anyone's pocket; it's insurance money.

For some years now, malpractice suits have been a method of squeezing money out of any mishap that could be uncovered or invented, and malpractice suits against physicians are presently epidemic. Medicine is and always will be an inexact science, where the unpredictable and the unknown responses of the human body to disease, medication, and treatment will forever perplex and dismay the most dedicated, careful, and skilled clinician. Not all operations will achieve their expected results because the capricious nature of healing of various tissues prohibits the guarantee of success in any procedure and will continue to do so in the foreseeable future. In theory, the surgeon is legally responsible for negligence, defined as carelessness plus injury or loss. In actuality, he is often sued (despite his best efforts and care) when an operation miscarries. As a rule, a legal inference of negligence does not arise merely because a surgical procedure had an unfavorable result. However, the doctrine in the law of torts known as *res ipsi loquitur* (the thing speaks for itself) has become the lawyer's mechanism for holding a physician accountable for any unfortunate result of careful treatment. The defendant doctor now finds himself in the position of being guilty unless he can prove himself innocent. This is somewhat illogical as the presumption of innocence is guaranteed in our system of justice for even the manifestly guilty until proven otherwise.

To say that this has had a chilling effect on practitioners of aesthetic surgery, where there is often a razor-edge line between a happy and an unhappy patient, would be an understatement. Because the specter of malpractice is assuming such haunting proportions, many conscientious surgeons who have spent their entire professional lives trying to perfect their field and their skills have been reluctant to undertake difficult cases for fear that an untoward result could trigger a suit.

Although it may be the insurance companies' money that is awarded, they make up for their losses by raising their premiums. No matter how high the premium, you may be sure that the physician will not pay for it. The patient will, pushing the already high cost of medicine to astronomical heights.

That physicians have contributed to this state of affairs is a belief shared by many. Much of the American public has an altered view of the present-day medical profession. Many people are scornful of doctors and feel that they are selfish and devote too much time to investments, stock market reports, business, and real estate. Part of the population refuses to be our allies for they feel that we have ceased to be their friends.

Granted there are a few bad apples in the barrel, but most physicians are honest, hardworking, and capable. Anyway what is so bad about a doctor becoming wealthy? In no other profession does an individual have to spend his best years and a great deal of money just preparing himself for his life's work. No other profession demands such skill and dedication, such long and bizarre hours, and such horrendous emotional expenditures. Most doctors deserve all the monetary rewards that come their way; they earn them.

Clearly, we must find a solution to this medico-legal morass or we will close the window on the development of new procedures, new methods of treatment, and even the investigation of new drugs. Naturally, our concern with safety should be paramount, but to expect a hundred percent guarantee under all circumstances is unrealistic. Without some calculated risks there is no action, no achievement, no progress. Without some risk the bright future of medicine and surgery will surely be relegated to some great twilight zone that knows neither success nor failure.

One solution to the problem would be a no-fault insurance program that would compensate an individual for injury or loss. This would decrease the need for litigation and do away with trials where sometimes the verdict of the jury is determined by their emotions and the capabilities of the attorney, rather than the facts of the case. This would not only lower costs considerably, but also would expedite compensatory awards when a patient was deserving of them.

Fewer suits would probably be initiated if an impartial

commission was created to investigate and determine if, indeed, there was a valid cause for a malpractice action. This would curtail the so-called frivolous or unwarranted lawsuit wherein an action is initiated to extort a settlement merely because that patient was unhappy with the physician or with the result of treatment. And most certainly, fewer justifiable suits would be filed if incompetent physicians were disciplined or removed from practice.

What about the other side of the scalpel? Who will continue to perform these operations? There are many specialty groups practicing these procedures, yet confusion reigns in the minds of patients seeking a reputable surgeon. One specialty advertises that only its group can adequately perform these surgeries. These specialists tell how rapidly they can process the cases and boast of how many different procedures they can perform during a surgical session. The common denominator of statements like these is that they are nonsensical or more likely, they are biased and self-serving for economic, competitive, or power-seeking reasons. They confuse motion with achievement and forget that the result is what's important—that the patient must live with his surgical result for a long time.

No one specialty has a monopoly on cosmetic surgery. Monopolies breed incompetence. Competition weeds out incompetent and inadequate surgeons in a field where artistry must be as great as accuracy. The mere existence of men of opposing specialties who successfully perform the work disproves the validity of these "one specialty only" claims. Let us hope we can part the curtain that separates us and become more understanding and tolerant of one another. In the final analysis, such an atmosphere will help and benefit the patient.

Overture for the Future

What of the future of cosmetic surgery? Is all this fuss over our looks really worth it? Will beauty be as important and as powerful in a future society? It certainly hasn't changed for thousands of years. In reality, we've only touched the surface. The cosmetic industry can vouch for that. What we are actually doing is investing in ourselves and that's one of the best stocks anyone can buy. It will be a plus for both men and women, but especially for women. Because men look at women in a much different way than women view men.

When a man looks at a woman, he generally sees her appearance, not her ability. For a woman and especially a beautiful woman, growing old in America can be a psychological death trip. Nature often bestows this favor with an iron hand, chaining its victims to a self-image whose emphasis is on looking good rather than on developing as a whole person. Time unravels this desolate betrayal.

Beauty has always been a desirable attribute, and it will be so in the foreseeable future. For like ugliness, it will remain a part of our lives and our environment. In fact, were beauty to be selectively inbred so that it became monotonous, there would always be someone or something just a little more beautiful to elicit excitement.

Although beauty is a stunning asset, there is no reason to get hysterical if you're not gorgeous. After all, beauty, like age, depends very much on one's point of view. Also, there are other subtle attributes which are more stirring and longer lasting—charm* and sex appeal. Neither guarantees happiness nor lasting romance, but they not only wear better, they also have little to do with looks or age. They are an acquired aura wrapped up in an engaging and electric personality. For an aging beauty, it is impossible to acquire charm via a face-lift. Although it may sound like a shallow cliché, true loveliness often comes from within. The wise man knows it and the mature woman is convinced of it. More often than not, it takes more than a cosmetic surgeon to turn an Eliza Doolittle into a fair lady.

In the near future, beauty and its design will become as essential a part of the training of cosmetic surgeons as is the mechanics of performing the procedures. The future cosmetic surgeon will receive art lessons as well as attend courses in cultural art. Not only will he be artistic, he will also be able to draw, and the step from easel to skin will not be a giant one. In this manner will specialists of cosmetic surgery continue to improve.

However, as no infallible guide exists for creating harmony out of disharmony, cosmetic surgeons will never operate with a foolproof system. Some patients will still become prisoners of their vanity, particularly when a case miscarries. Nor will

**The playwright, James M. Barrie, laid it on the line: "If you have it, you don't need anything else; and if you don't have it, it doesn't much matter what you have."*

cosmetic surgeons ever become social engineers. It is often difficult to stitch a formerly unattractive or aging person into the social fabric of the young and beautiful. Many people find it overwhelming when they cash in their years and deformities for the valued coin of attractiveness and youth. After surgery, many patients plunge into behavior far beyond their psychological depth. For some it does mark the first time that they can move about unnoticed, but for others their transformation produces a radical freedom from inhibition. Having lived a socially withdrawn life, these patients may be as naive and inexperienced in handling and judging situations as would an adolescent. Perhaps in the future, psychological evaluations of all persons requesting structural changes will be mandatory to help in their rehabilitation following surgery.

Ultimately, cosmetic surgery will be an integral part of everyday life. Despite genetic engineering, genetic copying, gene swapping and test-tube babies, deformities will still occur and people will still age. We arrive into the world wrinkled and most likely we will depart from the world wrinkled.

Endless situations will arise that may baffle and bewilder specialists in this field. However, they will continually adapt and respond to each new challenge with imaginative new technologies combined with a sharpened aesthetic sense. They will develop better methods to transform an ugly duckling into a beautiful swan, and they will refine ways to rejuvenate an old face and body. With certitude, I can state that the future of tomorrow's cosmetic surgeon is secure. He knows the best is yet to be.

Glossary

actinic
pertaining to the rays of the spectrum of light which produce chemical breakdown

aesthetic
pertaining to a sense of the beautiful

alopecia
baldness of varying degrees

analgesia
absence of the sense of pain in a limited area

analgesic
a drug that induces analgesia

anesthesia
total loss of consciousness, creating insensibility to pain

antigen
any substance which stimulates the production of antibodies

areola
the pigmented ring surrounding the nipple

atrophic
a wasting or reduction of a part which had previously reached mature size

auricular
pertaining to the ear

avascular
without blood

axillary
pertaining to the armpit

bilateral
pertaining to the right and left sides of a structure

biochemistry
the science dealing with the chemistry of living matter

blepharoplasty
cosmetic surgery of the eyelids

bridge

any ridge or spanlike structure; the nasal profile is often referred to as the nasal bridge

calorie

a unit of heat (adjective—caloric)

carbohydrate

an organic class of compounds represented by sugars, starches, and cellulose

carotene

a yellowish pigment of the skin

cartilage

gristle; a white, flexible semiopaque connective tissue comprising part of the skeleton (adjective—cartilaginous)

catalyst

a substance which increases the velocity of a chemical reaction

chemosurgery

the chemical removal of the superficial layers of the skin

circumferential

encircling or surrounding

collagen

connective tissue protein found in the dermis, and imparting suppleness, support, and elasticity to an organ

crown

the top part of the head

curet

a scoop-shaped surgical instrument for removing tissue from abdominal cavities

denervate

to interrupt the nerve supply to a part

dermabrasion

mechanical removal of the superficial skin surface

dermis

the true skin; the layer between the epidermis and the fatty tissue below (adjective—dermal)

dissection

the surgical cutting of tissues

diuretic
an agent that increases the volume of urine excreted

donor
the site from which a transplant or graft is taken

dorsum
the back; regarding the nose, it is synonomous with the nasal bridge

elastin
an essential protein in the dermis which helps to support and give elasticity to the skin

emollient
having the power of softening or relaxing living tissue; a soothing substance

epidermis
the outer layer of skin

excision
the surgical removal of tissue

fibrous
resembling fibers; containing fibroblasts, which are the essence of scar tissue

flap
a partially detached portion of skin and tissue which carries its own blood supply when transferred as a graft

flexion
the act of bending

follicle
the root of the hair

gene
the ultimate unit in the transmission of hereditary characteristics

gerontology
the branch of science that deals with the study of aging

graft
a living piece of tissue used to replace a defective part of the body

hemoglobin
the respiratory pigment of the red blood cells; can combine with and release oxygen

hypertrophy
an increase in the size of an organ, independent of natural growth (adjective—hypertrophic)

hypotensive
characterized by subnormal body blood pressure

hypothermic
characterized by subnormal body temperature

immutable
unchangeable

implant
a nonliving material placed within the body to repair a defect

incision
a cut into a tissue

keloid
an abnormal fibrous overgrowth of scar tissue characterized by itching and intermittent pain

labia minora
the inner fold of skin that surrounds the vaginal entrance

maceration
to soften or separate into parts by means of a solvent (adjective—macerated)

mastopexy
surgical reconstruction of a pendulous breast

melanin
the black or dark brown pigment of the body (adjective—melanoid)

mentoplasty
cosmetic surgery of the chin

motor nerve
that which causes motion

mucous membrane
the lubricating tissue lining an internal surface or an organ

nape
back of the neck

nasal
pertaining to the nose

navel

the belly button

nephropathic

causing damage to the kidney

orbital

the body cavity containing the eye (noun—orbit)

organ

a differentiated part of an organism adapted for a definite function

osmosis

the diffusion of fluid through a membrane

osteotomy

surgical cutting of bone

otoplasty

cosmetic surgery of the ears

oxyhemoglobin

oxidized hemoglobin; found in arterial blood

palate

the roof of the mouth

parameter

a determining factor

pathologies

any deviation from a healthy, normal, or efficient condition

placebo

a medicine having no pharmacologic effect, but given for the purpose of pleasing or humoring the patient; a sugar pill

postpartum

pertaining to the period of time following childbirth

preauricular

in front of the ear

prosthesis

the addition of an artificial part to augment or replace a defective or absent part of the body

recipient

the site that receives a graft or transplant

rejection
the casting out; in medicine, the loss of "take" of a graft or implant

rejuvenation
a renewal of youth

renal
pertaining to the kidney

resection
the surgical removal of part of an organ or tissue

retroussé
descriptive of a nasal profile having a minimal concavity to the bridge and a slight upward tilt to the tip

rhinoplasty
cosmetic surgery of the nose

rhytidoplasty
cosmetic surgery for the aging, sagging face; a face-lift

semilunar
crescent-shaped; like a half moon

semipermeable
ability of certain liquids to permeate or pass through a substance

serrating
to make notches; in otoplasty, notching or serrating weakens the cartilage, thus making it more pliable

serum
the clear yellow liquid that separates from the clot in the coagulation of blood

slough
a layer of dead tissue that separates from the surrounding living tissue

submental
the area immediately under the chin

tactile
pertaining to the sense of touch

temporal
pertaining to the temple

transplant

tissue removed from any portion of the body (or someone else's body) and placed in a different site

violaceous

bluish-purple color

Index